DELAVIER'S STRETCHING ANATOMY

Delavier's Stretching Anatomy

FRÉDÉRIC DELAVIER | JEAN-PIERRE CLÉMENCEAU | MICHAEL GUNDILL

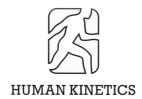

HUMAN KINETICS

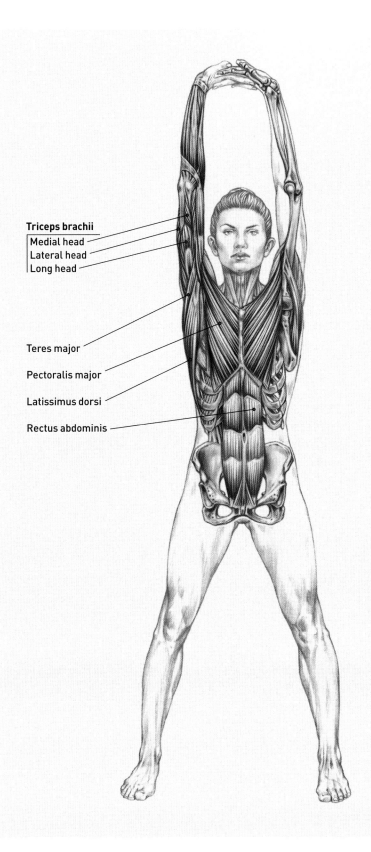

Triceps brachii
Medial head
Lateral head
Long head

Teres major

Pectoralis major

Latissimus dorsi

Rectus abdominis

INTRODUCTION

Why Stretching?

This book describes the most beneficial stretching exercises and explains how they can aid in your overall well-being.

Exercises That Reconnect You With Your Body

The secret to stretching lies in the simplicity of the movements. Since it is impossible to avoid stationary or stressful situations, you must learn how to stretch conscientiously and release tension. Otherwise, your muscles will freeze up and become stiff, which interferes with optimal circulation.

Stretching is not just a way to tone your body; it can also relieve stress by increasing your awareness of your body. Stretching, just like yoga, is a technique that increases your ability to handle emotional disruptions and improves your concentration.

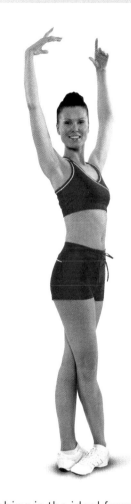

Stretching is the ideal form of exercise to help you discover how your body works and take control of your body. Stretching requires a confident attitude. It increases your confidence and makes you more comfortable with your body. It relaxes your muscles and increases circulation, all necessary for your well-being. In this way, it helps to release tension and eliminate aches and pains.

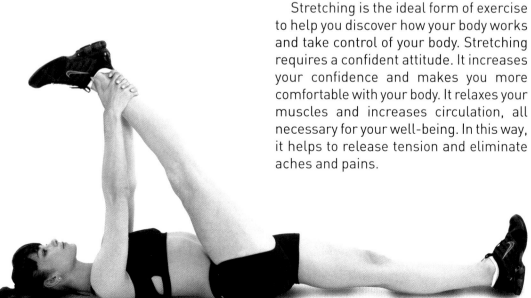

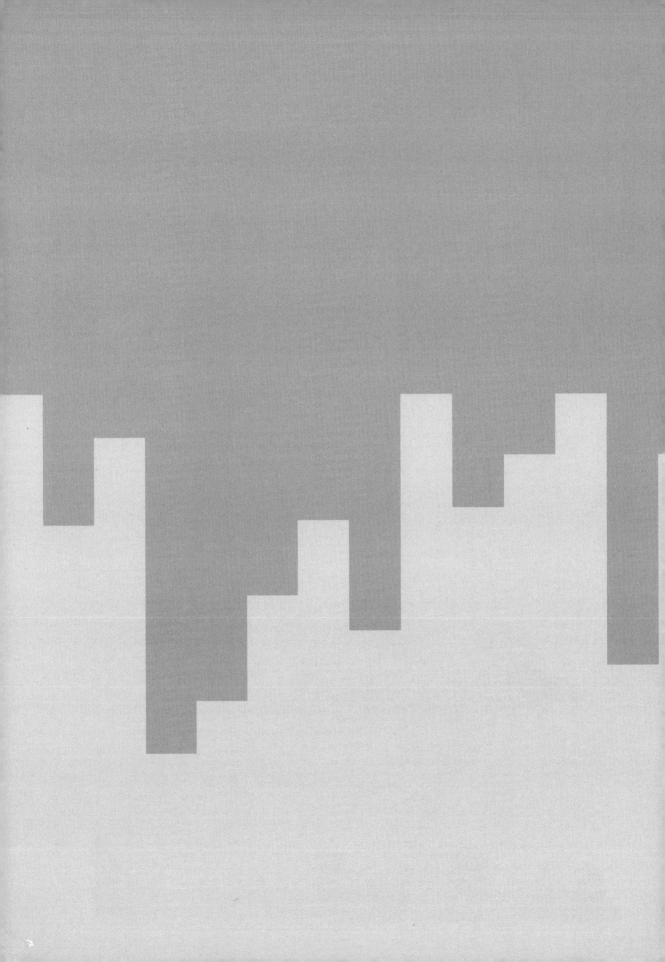

STRETCHING:
A USER'S MANUAL

A NATURAL METHOD BASED ON HOW YOUR BODY FEELS, NOT HOW HARD YOU PUSH

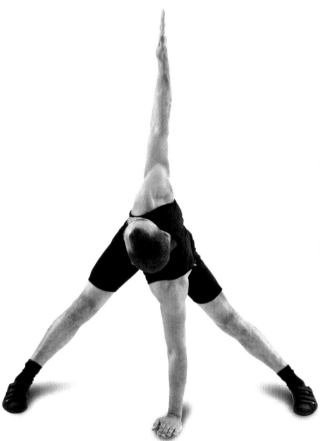

Stretching is essential for improving well-being, muscle tone, and flexibility. To achieve these benefits, you just need to do a few simple exercises regularly while focusing on your breathing.

BENEFITS OF STRETCHING

Stretching regularly will help you

→ relax both physically and mentally,
→ increase the flexibility of your muscles and tendons,
→ increase your range of motion,
→ improve your muscle tone,
→ develop cardiorespiratory endurance,
→ raise your fatigue threshold, and
→ prevent injuries and pain in both the muscles and the joints.

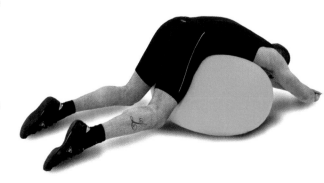

A GENTLE FORM OF EXERCISE

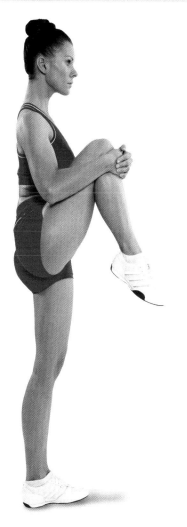

Stretching is a gentle exercise that involves no risk. It invites you to pay attention to your inner self instead of just worrying about your appearance. Stretching regularly will improve how you look as well as the way you move. You hold your head higher, your belly is flatter, your chest is open, and your legs are long. Gracefulness is the natural result of a supple body. The true beauty of your appearance has more to do with your physical balance than with your waist size, and it also has a lot to do with the flexibility of your muscles.

TYPES OF STRETCHING

There are various stretching techniques, but three main methods have proven effective.

1. STATIC STRETCHING

Static stretching is the most practiced stretching method. Because its purpose is to maintain the body in good physical form, static stretching is more appropriate for beginners and people who are not very active.

Static stretching relies on basic stretching movements and muscle contractions. These exercises, performed slowly over time, help you discover your deep (postural) muscles. They allow you to work your entire body while increasing awareness of your flexibility.

Muscles are lengthened using bending, extending, or twisting positions. These stretches must be done slowly so that the antagonistic muscles are not stimulated. Once you are comfortable in a stretched position, you hold the position for about 15 to 20 seconds to relax, lengthen, and oxygenate the muscle fibers.

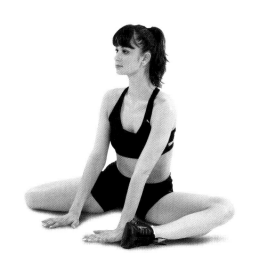

2. DYNAMIC STRETCHING

Dynamic stretching is often recommended in athletic training programs. It increases energy and power because it acts on the elasticity of muscles and tendons. It relies on swinging movements done with a certain amount of speed. The technique consists of swinging the legs or arms in a specific direction in a controlled manner without bouncing or jerky movements. The agonist muscle contracts rapidly, which lengthens the antagonist muscle, thereby stretching it.

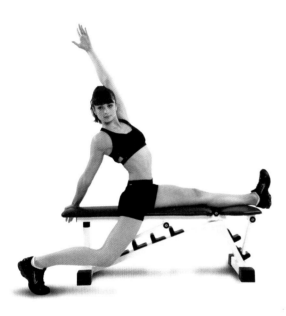

3. PNF STRETCHING

PNF stands for proprioceptive neuro-muscular facilitation. The PNF stretching technique is widely used in reeducation therapy. PNF stretching involves four steps:

1 Gradually stretch a muscle to its maximum.

2 Perform an isometric contraction for about 15 to 20 seconds (while still in the lengthened position).

3 Relax the muscle for about 5 seconds.

4 Restretch that same muscle for about 30 seconds.

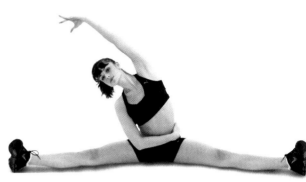

STRUCTURING A STRETCHING PROGRAM

→ A beginner program consists of 2 or 3 sets of each stretch. Each stretch should last 15 to 20 seconds. A complete program includes 5 to 7 stretches.

→ An intermediate program consists of 4 or 5 sets of each stretch; each stretch lasts 20 to 30 seconds. A complete program includes 6 to 8 stretches.

→ An advanced program consists of 5 or 6 sets of each stretch; each stretch lasts 20 to 45 seconds. A complete program includes 10 to 12 stretches.

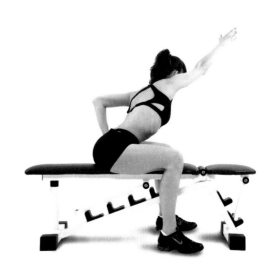

LEARN HOW TO BREATHE!

If you truly want to become more aware of your body, you must work on your breathing, oxygenation, and muscle relaxation. Your breathing during stretching should be calm and cadenced throughout the entire exercise so that your movements are slow and lengthened. You will achieve better oxygenation and muscle relaxation if your breathing is measured and progressive.

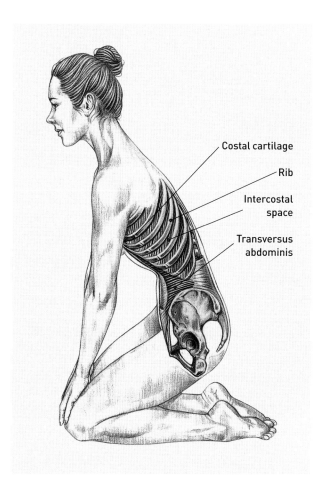

Costal cartilage

Rib

Intercostal space

Transversus abdominis

BREATHING AND RELAXATION

Relaxation achieved through stretching is not limited to muscle relaxation. When you detach yourself from your surroundings, you open your inner spirit. This allows you to focus on a single objective: finding your inner self by gathering your vital strength. Remember that, no matter what kind of stretching you do, your breathing should be normal (that is, slow and regular). Most important, you should never hold your breath while stretching because breathing provides oxygen to your muscles and releases tension.

FOR EFFECTIVE BREATHING

Most people do not use their full respiratory capacity. If you simply inhale and exhale deeply a few times, you will get a sense of how poorly people normally breathe. Learning to master your breathing and provide oxygen to your body will help you control your mind more easily and manage your emotions.

The saying "He forgot to breathe . . ." is not so far from the truth. So many illnesses, feelings of fatigue, and even episodes of fear or shyness can be resolved with a few deep breathing exercises! Lack of oxygen is also a factor in insomnia and stress.

INHALING AND EXHALING

At first, you need to become aware of your breathing: Is it rapid or calm? Is it deep or shallow? Are you breathing through your mouth or through your nose? Then, train yourself to breathe efficiently: calm, deep, and from the belly. Many people who are learning to stretch make the mistake of holding their breath to finish the exercise. This is the exact opposite of what you should do. It is better to inhale at the beginning of the stretch to oxygenate your muscles and then exhale while pushing, lifting, or pulling.

BREATHE DEEPLY, BUT FIND A NATURAL RHYTHM

Knowing how and with which part of the body to breathe allows you to optimize all stretches. In fact, you will decrease the impact of an exercise if you do it with chaotic and poorly controlled breathing. It is essential to avoid jerky inhalations and exhalations, no matter what kind of stretch you are doing.

ACTIVE BREATHING

Breathing is defined as the absorption of oxygen and the removal of carbon dioxide. An organism breathes using air pathways (the nose, the mouth, and the pharynx, whose role is to filter the inhaled air) and the lungs. Breathing can increase up to

20 times the normal rate during exercise. This increase brings in additional oxygen required by the organism and eliminates the carbon dioxide produced.

EXTERNAL BREATHING

The lungs are the primary organs for breathing, and they provide oxygen to the blood. In the lungs, gases are transferred between the air and the blood. The lungs' function is to provide sufficient oxygen for all vital processes and to eliminate metabolic waste products, such as carbon dioxide.

An organism regulates its rate of respiration as a function of need. The greater the effort, the faster the organism will breathe. During a stretching exercise, respiration increases progressively and then stabilizes.

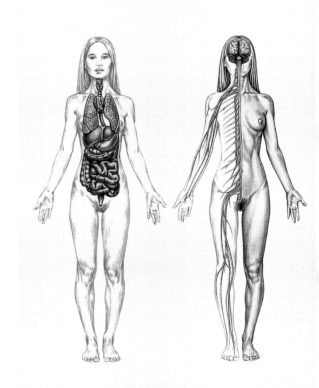

PULMONARY BREATHING

It is controlled by respiration centers in the brain. During stretching, respiration increases to provide for the energy needs of muscle cells. Two clearly differentiated types of breathing then begin: active respiration (inhaling through the nose) and passive respiration (exhaling through the mouth).

An organism mobilizes air through the action of respiratory muscles and the lungs. Inhalation is an active process primarily caused by the diaphragm, a muscle that separates the thorax from the abdomen. The levator costae and intercostal muscles contract, and the diaphragm lowers, which increases the volume of the rib cage. Since the pleura connect the lungs to the rib cage, the lungs follow the same movement.

During normal inhalation, the equivalent of a half liter of air enters the lungs, and three times that much enters during deep breathing! Exhalation is a passive phenomenon in which the levator costae and the intercostal muscles relax. The diaphragm moves back up and the lungs regain their initial volume.

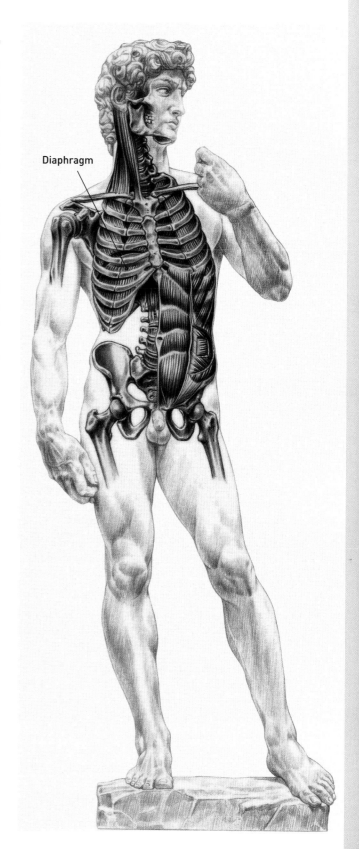

Diaphragm

WHY ATHLETES SHOULD STRETCH

Stretching is a natural gesture that maintains physical form and well-being. Instinctively, the first thing that we do when we wake up in the morning is stretch. Beyond this revitalizing aspect, stretching is also a good way to increase your athletic performance. In fact, flexibility is an important part of physical fitness.

STRETCHING HAS FIVE BENEFITS FOR ATHLETES

MAINTAIN OR INCREASE RANGE OF MOTION

Repetitive athletic movements can reduce your range of motion by tightening the muscles and tendons. A certain tension is required, especially in strength sports, but too much tension and a decreased range of motion can ultimately lead to injury and reduced quality of performance. Stretching regularly can prevent this problem. In certain sports and activities, like swimming or gymnastics, stretching must be done regularly to increase the range of motion in a joint when that range corresponds with increased performance.

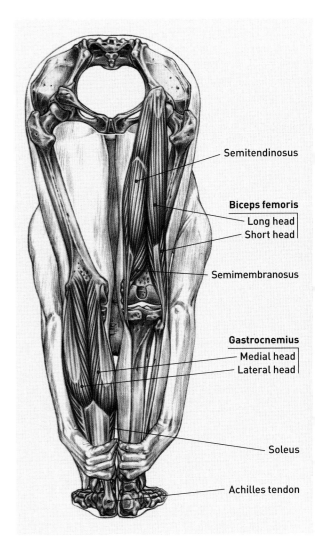

Semitendinosus

Biceps femoris
Long head
Short head

Semimembranosus

Gastrocnemius
Medial head
Lateral head

Soleus

Achilles tendon

INCREASE MUSCLE TONE

Stretching is a powerful signal to strengthen muscles. Using the muscle's strength in passive resistance, stretching accelerates the speed at which the proteins that make up the muscle fibers are synthesized. Your body gains muscle tone, strength, and resilience this way.

WARM UP BEFORE A WORKOUT

Stretching warms up the muscles, tendons, and joints, which prepares the body for physical exertion.

RELIEVE STRESS

Thanks to its euphoric and oxygenating effects, stretching minimizes stress that can tighten muscles (such as before a competition).

RELAX, RECUPERATE, AND PREVENT INJURIES

The majority of muscular efforts compress various joints as well as the spine. Stretching decompresses your back as well as your joints. This prevents injuries while accelerating recovery of the joints, tendons, and muscles.

TOO MUCH FLEXIBILITY CAN DIMINISH PERFORMANCE

For an athlete, flexibility is not the end in and of itself. It is certainly impressive to be flexible, but beyond a certain point, too much flexibility will diminish performance. It is better to find a good balance between muscle tension and flexibility. This balance was defined by the great Russian weightlifting masters: To prevent injuries and not hinder your performance, the muscle must be flexible enough to have a slightly greater range of motion than what is required by your sport, but not so much more that you would diminish performance by becoming like a rag doll whose joints move around too easily.

Conclusion: Stretching has the ability to increase or diminish performance levels. So you must be careful to use stretching properly.

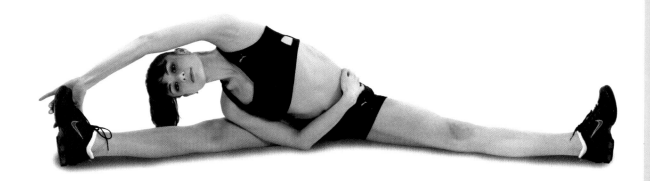

ATHLETES HAVE FOUR OPPORTUNITIES TO STRETCH

DURING WARM-UP

If you stretch out a rubber band for a few seconds, it will get warm. For this same reason, stretching warms up muscles and tendons. If you pull too hard on the rubber band, it will get too stretched and lose its strength. Even worse, it could break. The same thing can happen with muscles.

Warm-up stretching should always be done gently. In fact, medical research indicates that warm-ups with extended stretching can be associated with decreased performance caused by loss of muscle elasticity. Losing even a small amount of reactivity makes the muscle suddenly less explosive. This loss of performance lasts only a few hours, but that is enough time to interfere with a workout. Therefore, you should not push your stretches too far during your warm-up.

WHILE EXERCISING

When physical activity is fragmented (for example, in tennis, bodybuilding, soccer, or rugby), you can stretch during the breaks. At that moment, stretching can have two effects: In the best case, stretching allows you to regain muscle tone quickly by enhancing recuperation, which translates to an improvement in performance. In the worst case, stretching can accentuate the loss of muscle tone, which hastens fatigue.

These extremes can both be explained and are not as surprising as they first appear. They depend in large part on the degree of muscle fatigue achieved during exercise. It might even happen that stretching proves beneficial during the first part of a workout and then counter-productive at the end of the workout. The opposite can also happen. The advantage of stretching is that you can immediately feel any benefits or damaging effects. So you should not feel that you have to stretch during every workout. Even if some people love to do it, it in no way benefits every person in every situation.

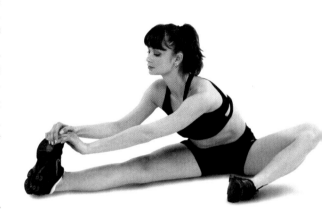

IMMEDIATELY AFTER A WORKOUT

This is the best time to stretch. In fact, no matter the results, you will not suffer from the potential temporary decrease in performance. Ideally, you should stretch the muscles you just used because, at that moment, they are still really warm and they need to recover. However, keep in mind the rule stressed thus far: Being too flexible can decrease your performance in the long run. Simply maintain a good range of motion in order to prevent injuries.

BETWEEN WORKOUTS

Stretches can be used to accelerate recovery between workouts. Stretching can reinforce the muscle-regeneration process.

Stretching has two advantages: It is not very tiring and it can be done at home without the need for any equipment.

But be careful not to overdo it! Past a certain point, too many sets of stretches can tire out the muscle instead of helping it to recover. A good amount of work for a muscle group is 2 to 4 sets of static stretches held for 15 to 20 seconds.

The second problem inherent in this strategy is that you are working the muscle when it is cold, which could be dangerous. So remember to warm up a little before you stretch and gradually increase the length of your stretches.

HOW AN ATHLETE SHOULD STRETCH

There are two primary techniques for athletic stretching.

STATIC STRETCHING

Static stretching consists of holding a stretch for 10 seconds to 1 minute. The degree of stretch can be from very light to rather strong depending on your objective.

Advantage: Practiced in a controlled and progressive manner, static stretching is very unlikely to cause an injury.
Disadvantage: This type of stretching is most likely to cause a decrease in performance when done just before a workout.

DYNAMIC STRETCHING

Dynamic stretching consists of pulling more or less forcefully on a muscle using small, repetitive movements for 10 to 20 seconds. This type of stretching resembles plyometrics because it plays on the stretch–relax cycle (or elasticity) and causes a reflex contraction. The goal of the small movements is to force the muscle to lengthen more than it would do so naturally.

Advantage: Dynamic stretching is the least likely to cause a decrease in performance when done before a workout, so long as the muscle does not tear. But you must be extremely careful when doing this type of stretching because it can cause injuries.
Disadvantage: This kind of stretching is the most likely to cause injury.

Generally, you should do 1 to 3 sets of stretches per muscle group. Then the only thing you as the athlete need to do is determine which muscles you wish to stretch depending on your sport as well as your personal needs. To help you in this task, see the variety of programs in the third part of this book (page 127).

BREATHING DURING STRETCHING

Breathing affects muscle tone in these ways:

→ Muscles can express their full power only when you hold your breath.
→ They are a little weaker when you exhale.
→ They are weakest during inhalation.

Holding your breath during a stretch will stiffen the muscle. So when stretching, you must relax your body. Inhale calmly for an extended period to make the muscle lose most of its resistance. You should therefore synchronize your breath with the stretch and exhale during the most intense part of the stretch.

STRETCHING UNILATERALLY

You will notice that you are always more flexible when you stretch one limb at a time than when you stretch the left and right sides at the same time.

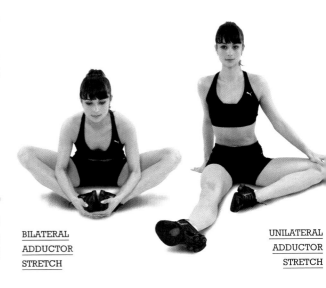

BILATERAL
ADDUCTOR
STRETCH

UNILATERAL
ADDUCTOR
STRETCH

BILATERAL
QUADRICEPS STRETCH

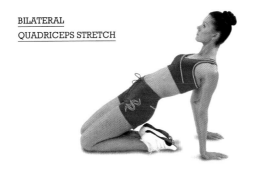

UNILATERAL
QUADRICEPS STRETCH

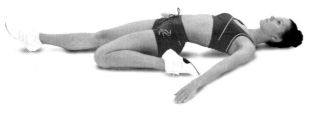

If you are an athlete looking to increase your range of motion quickly, you should do more unilateral stretches than bilateral stretches.

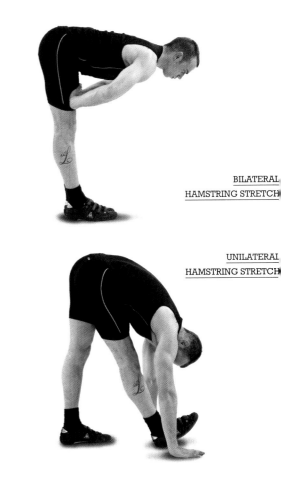

BILATERAL
HAMSTRING STRETCH

UNILATERAL
HAMSTRING STRETCH

   This physiological peculiarity shows the role of the nervous system in stretching. You might think that only muscle and tendon flexibility determines range of motion. But bilateral stretches show that the nervous system's protective blockage begins much sooner bilaterally than unilaterally. The range of motion is therefore more restricted.

STRETCHING TO PREVENT PROBLEMS ASSOCIATED WITH SPORTS

You often hear that playing sports is good for your health. Paradoxically, athletes often have annoying problems such as cramps, stiff muscles, muscle spasms, pulled muscles, and even muscle tears and ruptures. Stretching regularly can reduce the frequency of these problems.

CRAMPS

Cramps, which often happen to athletes, are due to an involuntary and forceful contraction of a muscle. The pain goes away after a few minutes and sometimes after just a few seconds. Cramps are often caused by poor hydration, a lack of magnesium or sodium, an insufficient workout, an inappropriate movement, or an incorrect position.

Nighttime cramps have been linked to deficiencies in magnesium, B-vitamins, and calcium. They can also be caused by a narrowing of the arteries if they are coated with plaque, by excessive alcohol intake, or by diabetes-related problems. To eliminate a cramp, stretch the cramped muscle to force it to relax immediately.

STIFF MUSCLES

Stiff muscles are diffuse muscle pains that often affect several muscle groups at the same time. They usually occur the day after or two days after intense muscular effort and can last from three days to more than one week. Stretching regularly before and after workouts will eventually prevent muscle stiffness. However, in the short term, stretching can actually cause stiff muscles.

⚠ Warning!
Stiffness can occur in muscles that are not accustomed to being stretched.

When you perform a new exercise, you stretch the junction between the tendon and the muscle in an unfamiliar way. This stretching can damage the muscle fibers, which may cause stiffness. This is why beginning a new stretching program can cause muscle stiffness. However, this stiffness will act as a vaccine against future muscle stiffness. If you do the stretches again a few days later, you will have practically no stiffness, which demonstrates the human body's extraordinary ability to adapt.

MUSCLE SPASMS

Spasms manifest with the presence of a hard and painful knot in the muscle. Unlike cramps, which start and stop quickly, spasms can take days to resolve. The muscles are very stiff and locked up. Muscle spasms are a symptom of fatigue and injury. Athletes who do not truly master their physical capabilities can experience muscle spasms as a result of excessive effort.

A good stretching program should focus first on problem areas in order to prevent muscle spasms.

PULLED MUSCLES

Pulled muscles are the first stage of serious muscle problems. A pulled muscle occurs when the muscle is stretched too forcefully and sometimes beyond its normal length.

The fibers are not affected, but the connective tissue is stretched. Only rest will help resolve this rather intense pain. Stretching is the best way to prevent pulled muscles.

MUSCLE TEARS

Like a pulled muscle, a tear affects the connective tissue. It occurs when you continue to push yourself too hard with tired or even injured muscles. Torn muscles are the nemesis of high-level athletes because the injury can interrupt a sport season for as long as six months.

⚠ Warning!
If the muscle is poorly rehabilitated or used before it is completely healed, a second tear can then cause serious problems.

Just as for pulled muscles, stretching is the best way to prevent tears.

MUSCLE RUPTURE

Muscle rupture is damage to a large group of fibers inside the muscle. Athletes call this injury a case of going too far. You have nearly finished your workout and your muscles are feeling tired, but despite that you want to do a little bit more, beyond your limit. Unfortunately, your tired muscles do not agree!

The solution: Rest and medical treatment involving ionization or laser therapy. A progressive bodybuilding program combined with stretching is the most effective way to protect against ruptures. For more about this, see *The Strength Training Anatomy Workout* by Frédéric Delavier (Human Kinetics).

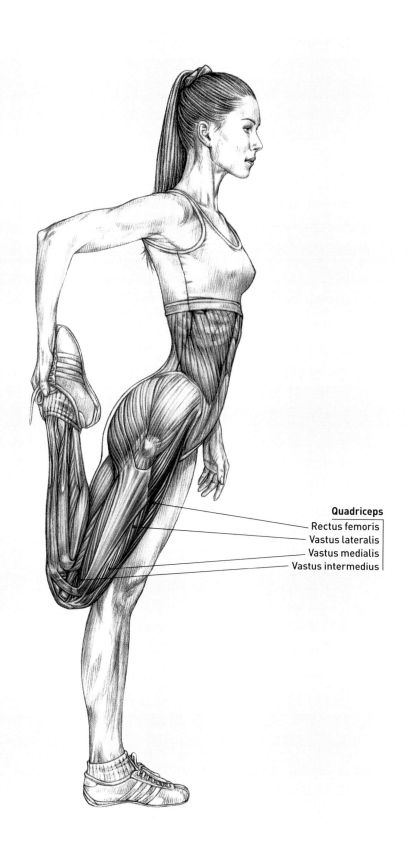

Quadriceps
Rectus femoris
Vastus lateralis
Vastus medialis
Vastus intermedius

THE STRETCHES

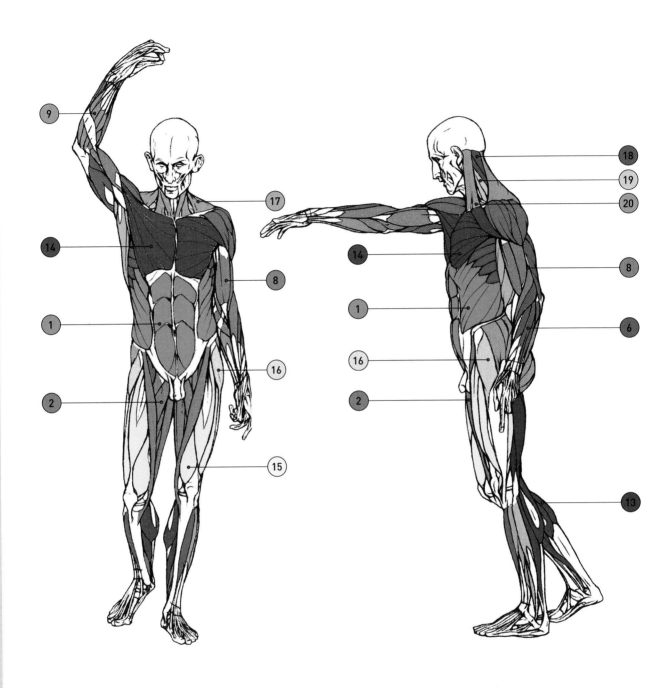

1. **Abdominals** p. 58
2. **Adductors** p. 111
3. **Latissimus dorsi** p. 71
4. **Shoulders** p. 34
5. **Triceps** p. 50

6. **Wrist extensors** p. 50
7. **Buttocks** p. 87
8. **Biceps** p. 50
9. **Wrist flexors** p. 50
10. **Shoulder blade fixators** p. 71

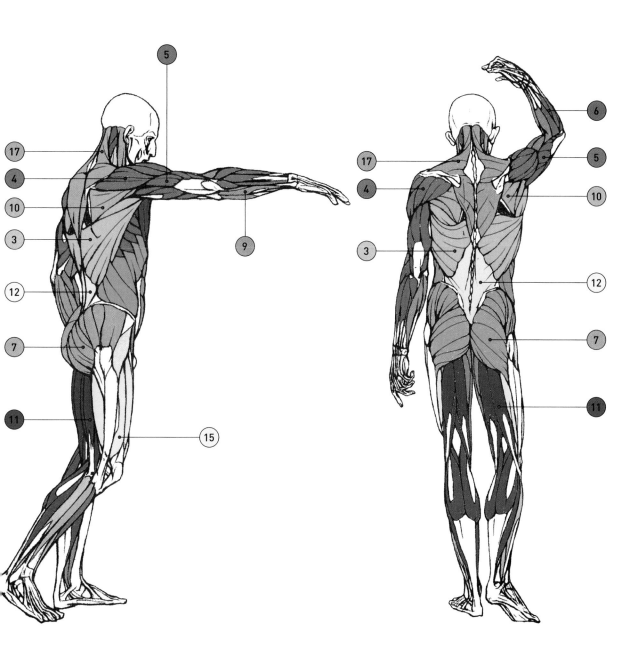

STRETCHES FOR THE NECK

The neck is subject to a lot of abuse not only during the day but also at night. How many times have you woken up with pain in your neck or even torticollis (twisted neck)? By stretching and strengthening your neck muscles while lightly decompressing your cervical vertebrae, a stretching program can help prevent these painful episodes that can severely restrict your movement.

The neck muscles have two purposes: They ensure flexibility in the neck (they allow you to turn your head from one side to the other and to look up and down), and they protect the integrity of the cervical vertebrae (the cervical vertebrae suffer abuse caused by the great flexibility of the neck and the head's heavy weight). It is therefore essential to maintain strength in these protective muscles.

The top of the trapezius muscles should not be neglected, either, because they support the neck muscles in their protective role.

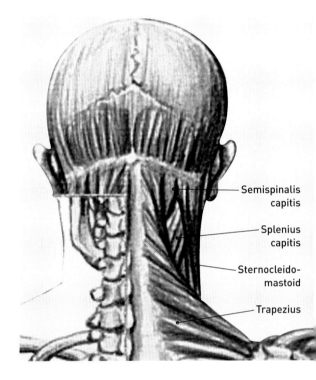

- Semispinalis capitis
- Splenius capitis
- Sternocleido-mastoid
- Trapezius

⚠ Warning!

Since the cervical vertebrae are small but have great mobility, it is easy to injure them. The purpose of stretching is to strengthen the neck muscles so that they can best protect the integrity of the cervical vertebrae. However, you must not forget that you can also injure your cervical vertebrae though excessive, abrupt, or improper stretching. You must stretch your neck in a very controlled manner so that you do not compress the cervical vertebrae you are trying to protect.

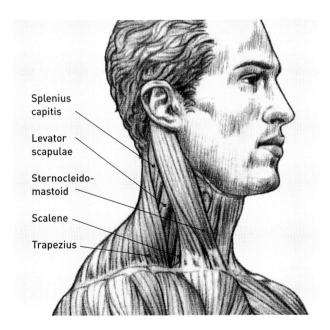

- Splenius capitis
- Levator scapulae
- Sternocleido-mastoid
- Scalene
- Trapezius

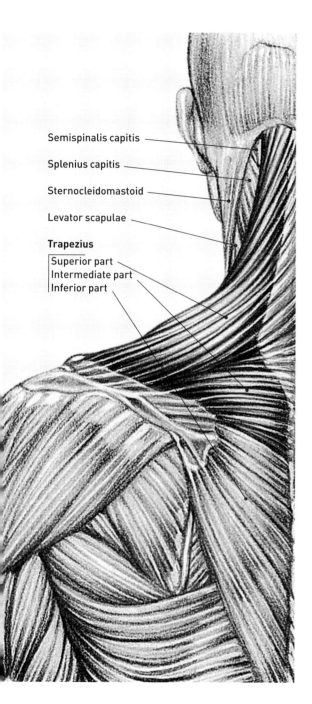

Semispinalis capitis

Splenius capitis

Sternocleidomastoid

Levator scapulae

Trapezius

Superior part
Intermediate part
Inferior part

A complete stretching program for the neck must include an exercise that works the muscles located in these areas:

→ Side of the neck (rotator muscles)
→ Back of the neck (extensor muscles)
→ Front of the neck (flexor muscles)

SIDE OF THE NECK

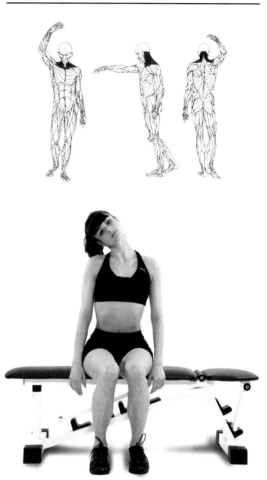

This exercise stretches the sides of the neck.

Sit on a bench with your feet flat on the floor and your torso very straight with your arms hanging by your sides. Lightly contract your buttocks so that you do not compensate with your lumbar spine, and then slowly tilt your head to the right side as far as you can. Take the time to inhale and exhale slowly and regularly throughout the exercise. Once you have stretched the right side, repeat the exercise on the left side.

ADVANCED VERSION

This neck stretch is similar to the preceding one, but it is more intense. The starting position is the same. To increase the intensity of the stretch, place the palm of your hand on the ear of the opposite side. Then, slowly push with your hand so that your head comes as close to your shoulder as possible. Hold the position for a few seconds. Be sure to breathe throughout the exercise.

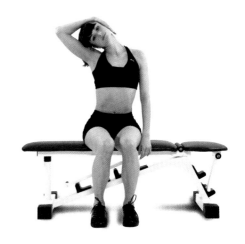

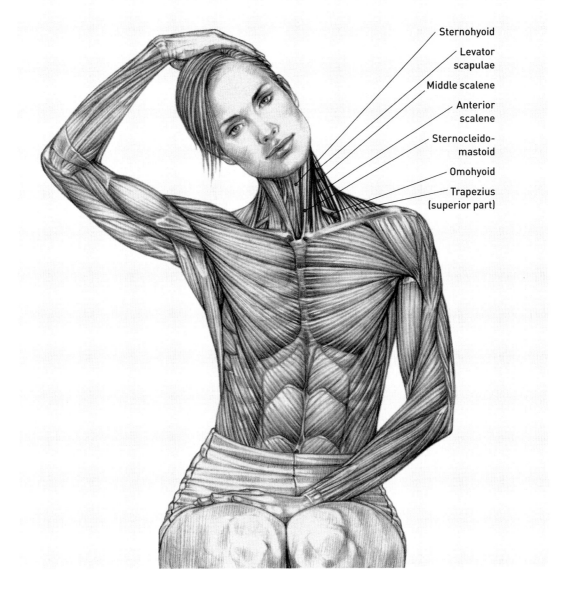

Sternohyoid

Levator scapulae

Middle scalene

Anterior scalene

Sternocleido-mastoid

Omohyoid

Trapezius (superior part)

VERSION WITH ONE ARM BEHIND YOUR BACK

Stand with your legs slightly apart, back very straight, and one arm behind your back. Grab the wrist with your other hand and pull slowly out and toward your arm so that you can feel a stretch in your deltoid and trapezius muscles. If you tilt your head to the opposite side of the shoulder you are stretching, you will accentuate the stretch in the trapezius and the neck muscles. You will also stretch the deep and complex muscles on the edge of the cervical spine as well as the scalenes and the sternocleidomastoid.

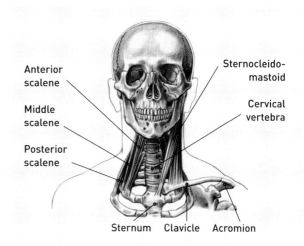

Anterior scalene

Middle scalene

Posterior scalene

Sternocleido-mastoid

Cervical vertebra

Sternum   Clavicle   Acromion

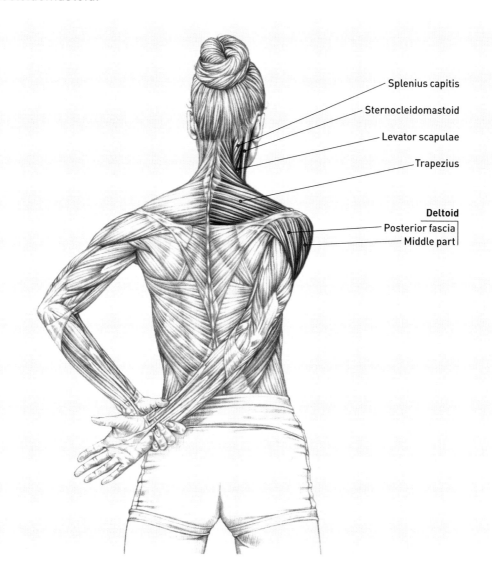

Splenius capitis

Sternocleidomastoid

Levator scapulae

Trapezius

Deltoid
Posterior fascia
Middle part

SIDE OF THE NECK

BACK OF THE NECK

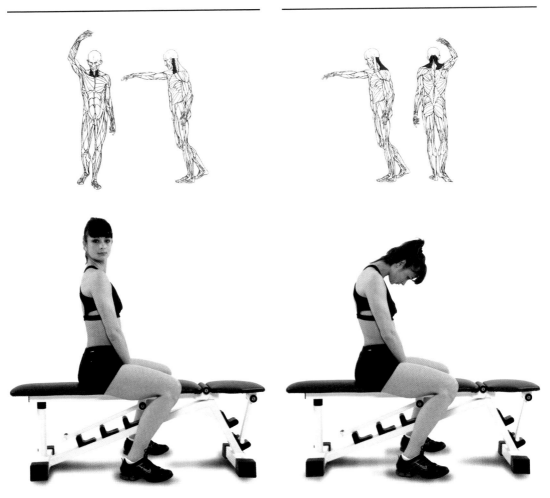

This exercise allows you to stretch the whole side of the neck.

Straddle a bench with your torso straight, your feet flat on the floor, and your hands resting on the bench inside your thighs. Slowly turn your head to the right without moving your shoulders. Hold this position for about 30 seconds, breathing slowly and regularly, and then repeat on the left side.

This exercise stretches the back of the neck.

Straddle a bench with your feet flat on the floor for stability and to avoid compensating with your lumbar spine. Put your hands inside your thighs on the bench and then lean your head forward while keeping your torso straight. Hold this position for about 30 seconds while breathing slowly and regularly.

FRONT OF THE NECK

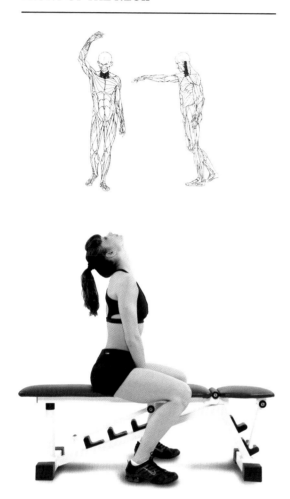

This exercise stretches the front of the neck.

Straddle a bench with your torso straight, legs bent, and feet flat on the floor for stability. Put your hands on the bench on the inside of your thighs. Slowly tilt your head backward while gently clenching your jaw. Hold this position for 15 to 20 seconds, breathing normally throughout the stretch.

STRETCHES FOR THE SHOULDERS AND CHEST

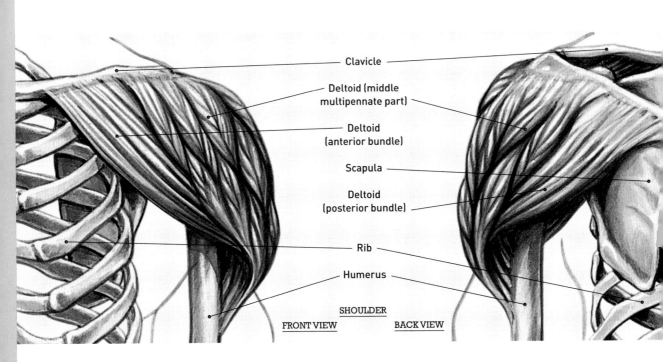

Clavicle

Deltoid (middle multipennate part)

Deltoid (anterior bundle)

Scapula

Deltoid (posterior bundle)

Rib

Humerus

SHOULDER

FRONT VIEW   BACK VIEW

More than one-third of the adult population will suffer from shoulder problems at some point in their lives. These problems primarily stem from minor to severe tears in the rotator cuff muscles. These occur even more frequently in athletes, especially in activities involving repetitive shoulder motions such as swimming, tennis, and throwing sports.

position. Without these muscles, the shoulder joint would dislocate immediately during the slightest movement.

It is easy to see how excessive use of the deltoid could easily lead to injuries in the stabilizing muscles in the shoulder. These injuries are even more common because these four protector muscles are rather small. Of the four muscles, the infraspinatus is the most heavily used and the most fragile. This is why you should tone it using specific stretches.

TO PREVENT SHOULDER PAIN, STRETCH THE INFRASPINATUS

The infraspinatus is one of the four muscles that form the rotator cuff. The rotator cuff is a quartet of muscles that enclose the shoulder joint to keep it in

PREVENTING SHOULDER PAIN IN ATHLETES

Sports that require a lot of shoulder movement can easily cause pain in the deltoid

ROTATOR CUFF MUSCLES,
FRONT VIEW

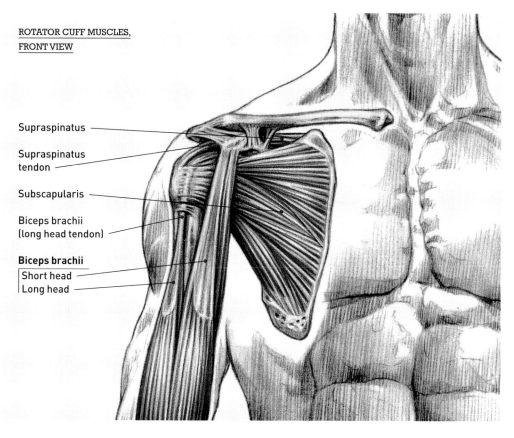

Supraspinatus

Supraspinatus
tendon

Subscapularis

Biceps brachii
(long head tendon)

Biceps brachii
Short head
Long head

ROTATOR CUFF MUSCLES,
BACK VIEW

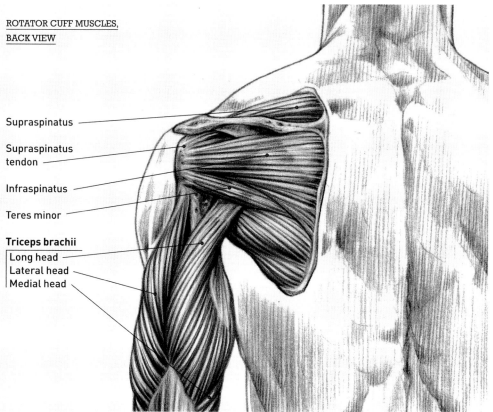

Supraspinatus

Supraspinatus
tendon

Infraspinatus

Teres minor

Triceps brachii
Long head
Lateral head
Medial head

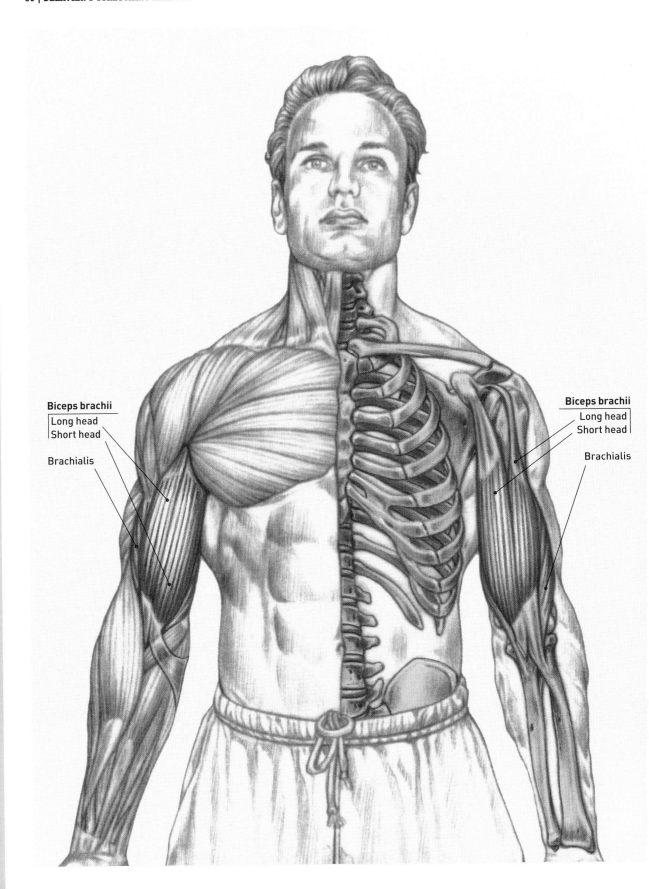

Biceps brachii
Long head
Short head

Brachialis

Biceps brachii
Long head
Short head

Brachialis

muscle. This often happens in throwing sports (basketball, volleyball, handball, shot put), combat sports, tennis, nautical sports, swimming, arm wrestling, climbing, golf, and bodybuilding. To prevent this pain, you need to maintain stability in the joint and tone the supporting muscles (that is, the back of the shoulder, the infraspinatus, and the lower trapezius).

Be specific!

Some activities, like swimming, require great flexibility in the shoulders to facilitate movement. However, other sports, and strength sports in particular, require a certain amount of stiffness in the shoulders to gain power and rigidity for movement.

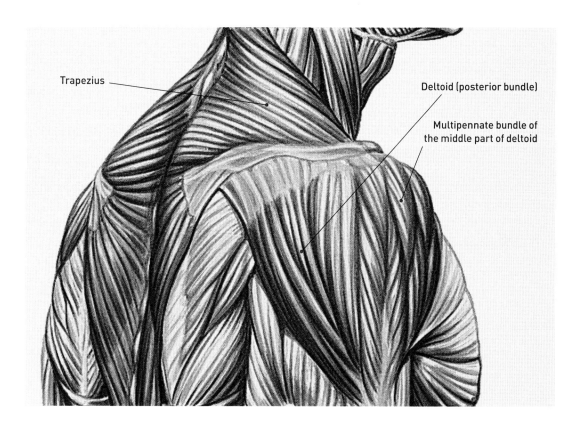

Trapezius

Deltoid (posterior bundle)

Multipennate bundle of the middle part of deltoid

⚠ Warning!

The muscles in the front and the back of the shoulder, as well as their tendons, play an important role in stabilizing the scapulohumeral joint (the arm joint on the shoulder blade). Because of its molecular structure (which is very resistant to abrasion), the tendon of the long head of the biceps was not designed to become very flexible. Stretching it too far could result in an injury. In addition, if the shoulder itself is too flexible, it could dislocate too easily during an abrupt movement or a fall.

HOW TO PROTECT THE INFRASPINATUS

As an athlete, you should stretch the infraspinatus in two ways: during warm-up and after working out.

→ **During warm-up:** Every workout session should begin with two or three light infraspinatus stretches. This warm-up prevents the muscle from being too cold when you begin your workout. In addition, this kind of regular stretching will provide deep strengthening to prevent injuries.

→ **After a workout:** When the warm-up is not enough, or if you feel that your shoulder is unstable, more intense training is necessary. Most people realize that they need to work on the infraspinatus only when their shoulders start hurting, but it is better to figure this out later than never. In this case, perform 3 to 5 sets of infraspinatus stretches at the end of your workouts. This additional work does not eliminate the need for the warm-up stretches.

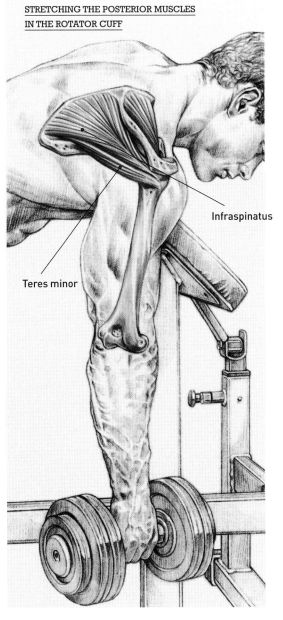

STRETCHING THE POSTERIOR MUSCLES IN THE ROTATOR CUFF

Infraspinatus

Teres minor

1

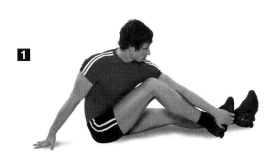

2

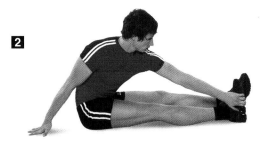

STRETCHING THE INFRASPINATUS

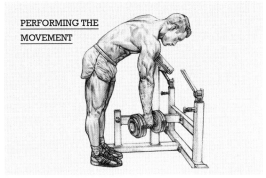

PERFORMING THE MOVEMENT

FRONT OF THE SHOULDER AND CHEST

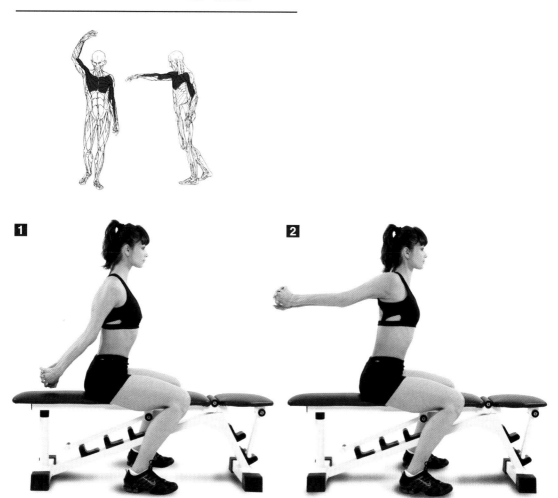

This exercise stretches the front of the shoulder and the chest muscles.

Straddle a bench with your legs bent, feet flat on the floor, and torso straight. Clasp your hands behind your back with your palms together **1**. Slowly raise your arms as high as you can **2**, being careful not to force it and not to arch your lumbar spine. Hold this position for 20 seconds while breathing regularly, and then relax.

VERSION WITH PALMS FACING BEHIND YOU

VERSION WITH PALMS FACING OUT

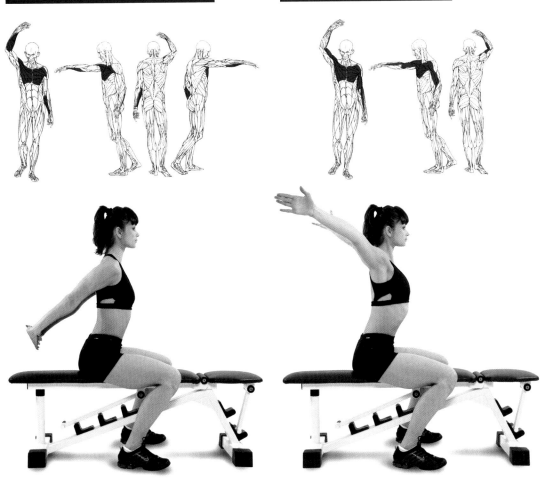

Straddle a bench with your legs bent, feet flat on the floor, and torso straight. Put your arms behind your back and clasp your hands with your palms facing behind you. Hold this position for 20 seconds while breathing regularly, then relax. This stretch is different from the previous one because of the position of your hands: Since they are facing out, you are also stretching your finger joints.

Straddle a bench with your legs bent, feet flat on the floor, and torso straight. Put your arms in back so they're raised slightly above your shoulders with your palms facing out and your shoulder blades pulled together. Hold this position for 15 to 20 seconds while breathing slowly and regularly. This exercise stretches the shoulders.

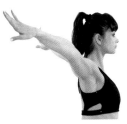

This version is similar to the previous one except that the palms are turned inward to better isolate the stretch in the shoulders.

ANTERIOR BUNDLE OF THE DELTOIDS

This movement primarily works the deltoids.

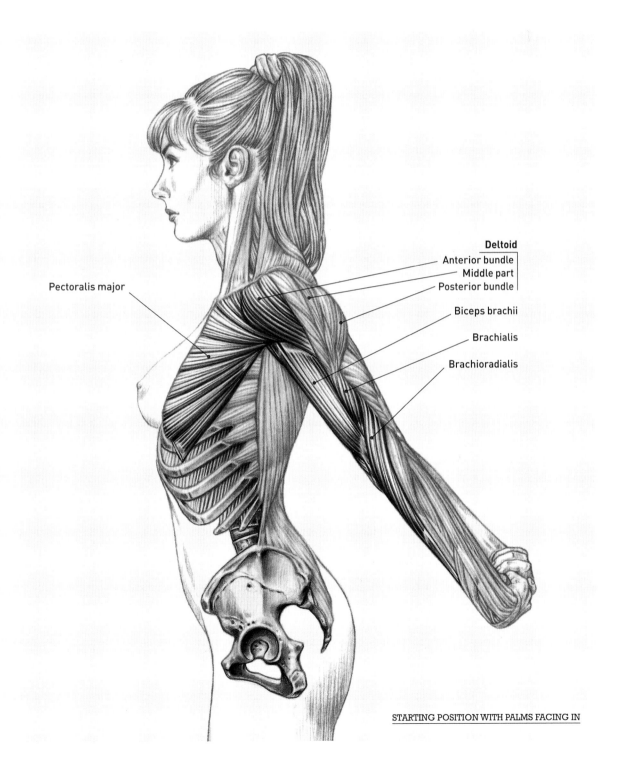

Pectoralis major

Deltoid
Anterior bundle
Middle part
Posterior bundle

Biceps brachii

Brachialis

Brachioradialis

STARTING POSITION WITH PALMS FACING IN

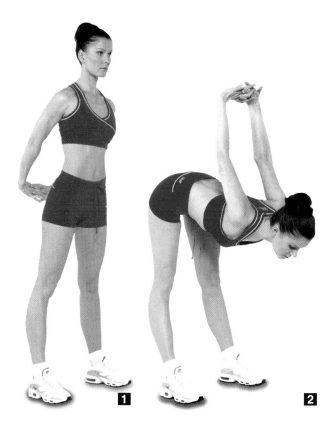

1

2

ADVANCED VERSION USING A SUPPORT

Stand near a chair with your hands clasped behind your back and your palms facing in **1**. Lower yourself until you can put your hands on the back of the chair, then continue lowering yourself while leaning forward **2**. Go forward by moving your pelvis forward. The farther you push your pelvis forward, the more intense the stretch **3**. When you find the position that works for you, stay there for 15 to 20 seconds. Do this exercise gently, without forcing anything, and be sure to breathe. You can also put a towel on the back of the chair to avoid bruising your wrists.

Begin the exercise standing up with your legs straight, feel parallel, and hands clasped behind your butt—hands facing out **1** or facing in (see page 41). Bend your torso forward while keeping your arms straight above your shoulders **2**. Exhale and inhale slowly throughout the exercise. Hold the position for about 30 seconds and then gently bend your knees and roll up through your back, which will prevent any pulling on your lumbar spine. This is one of the best flexibility exercises. It primarily works the deltoids so you can have elegant posture with your shoulders pulled back.

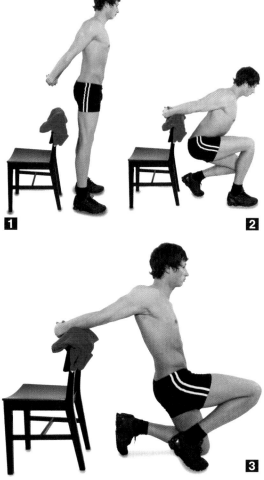

1

2

3

ADVANCED VERSION USING A BATON

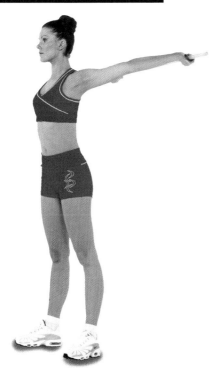

Stand with your feet apart and your hands holding the ends of a baton above your head. With straight arms, make an arc to bring the baton behind your back. Hold this position for 15 to 20 seconds while breathing slowly and regularly.

BACK OF THE SHOULDER, TRAPEZIUS, AND RHOMBOIDS

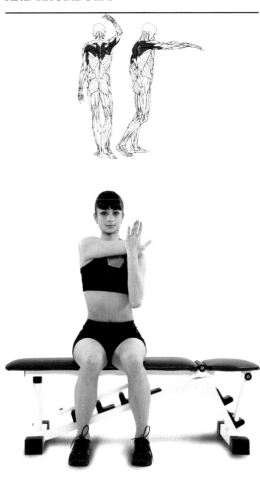

This exercise increases flexibility in the back of the shoulder, the middle of the trapezius muscles, and the rhomboid muscles.

Sit on a bench with your torso straight, legs slightly apart, and feet flat on the floor. Bend your right arm and bring it across your chest at shoulder level. Place your left hand on your right elbow. Push gently and hold this position for about 30 to 40 seconds, breathing slowly and regularly. Then repeat the exercise on the left side.

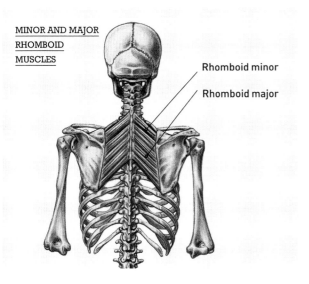

MINOR AND MAJOR RHOMBOID MUSCLES

Rhomboid minor

Rhomboid major

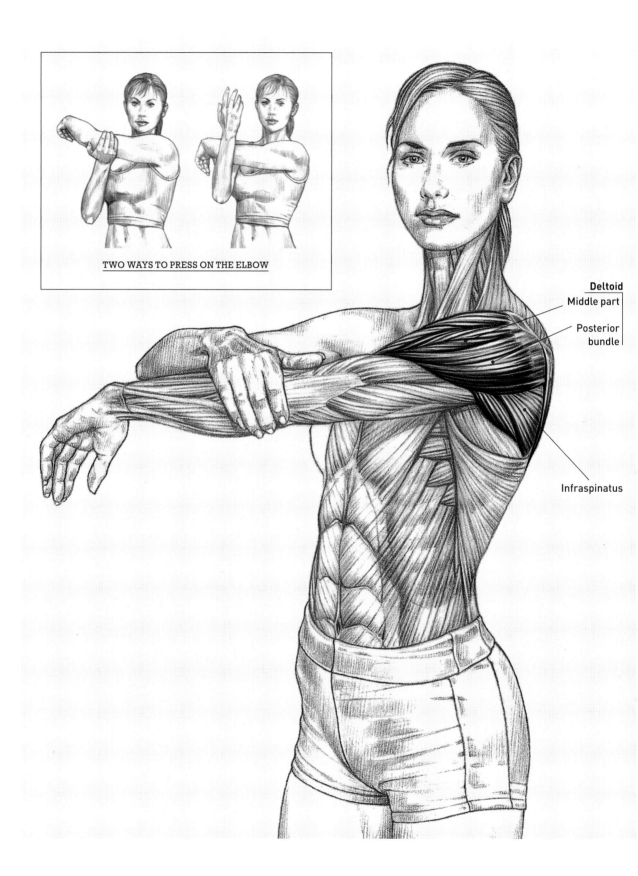

TWO WAYS TO PRESS ON THE ELBOW

Deltoid
Middle part

Posterior
bundle

Infraspinatus

BILATERAL VERSION

VERSION USING A SUPPORT

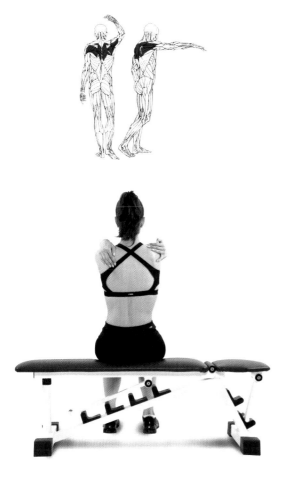

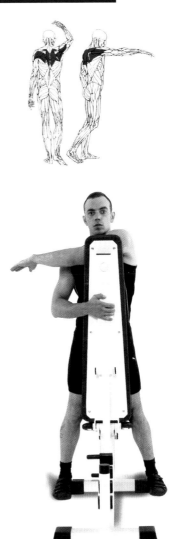

Sit on a bench with your torso straight and feet firmly on the floor for good posture. Put the palm of each hand on the opposite shoulder, being careful to keep your elbows horizontal. Pull gently and simultaneously to stretch your shoulders thoroughly. Hold the position for 15 to 20 seconds while you inhale and exhale slowly and regularly.

Stand with your torso straight. Rest one hand on a support and bend the other arm across your chest at shoulder level. Hold for a few seconds to get a good shoulder stretch, and be sure to breathe slowly and regularly. Then repeat the stretch on the other side.

SHOULDER AND TRICEPS

ADVANCED VERSION

This exercise stretches the deltoids and triceps.

Sit on a bench with your torso straight, legs slightly apart, and feet flat on the floor. Lift one arm up and bend it behind your head. With your other hand, reach behind your back and grasp the fingers of the other hand. Hold the stretch for 30 to 50 seconds to get a good stretch in the entire shoulder. For this stretch, pull your shoulder blades together so your torso stays very straight. Once you have stretched the first side, repeat the stretch on the other side.

Sit on a bench with your torso straight, legs slightly apart, and feet flat on the floor. Lift one arm up and bend it behind your head. With your other hand, reach behind your back and grasp the fingers of the other hand. Gently bend your torso away from the side of your raised arm. Hold this position for about 30 seconds and then repeat the stretch on the other side. This version stretches the shoulders, triceps, obliques, and latissimus dorsi.

CHEST AND FRONT OF SHOULDER

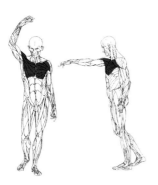

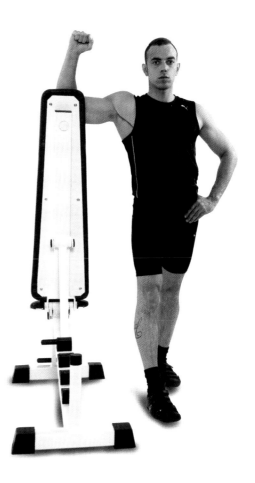

This stretch is for all the chest muscles and the front of the shoulder.

Stand next to a tall support with one leg in front of the other and the outside hand on your waist. Bend your inside arm at a right angle and raise it to shoulder level. Gently press your arm against the support. Hold the stretch for 20 to 30 seconds, and be sure to inhale and exhale regularly. Repeat the stretch on the other side.

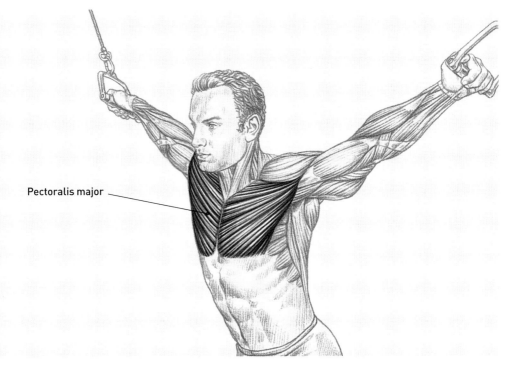

Pectoralis major

CHEST

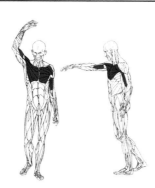

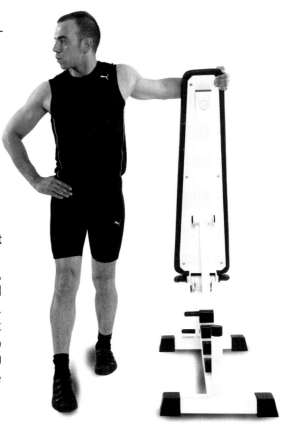

This exercise stretches all the chest muscles.
Stand with one leg in front of the other, right hand on your waist, and left hand at shoulder level against a tall support. Your left arm should be slightly bent. Twist gently to the right and turn your head to the right. Hold the position for about 30 seconds and breathe slowly. Repeat the exercise on the other side.

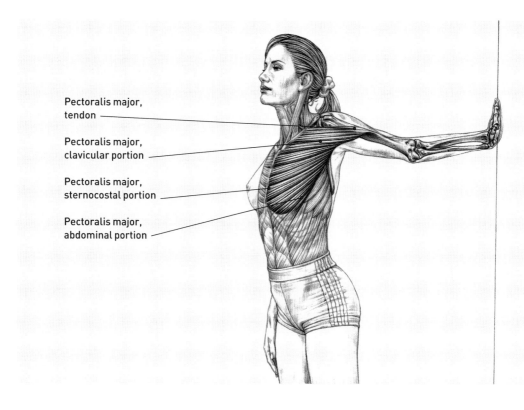

Pectoralis major, tendon

Pectoralis major, clavicular portion

Pectoralis major, sternocostal portion

Pectoralis major, abdominal portion

VERSION WITH STRAIGHT ARM

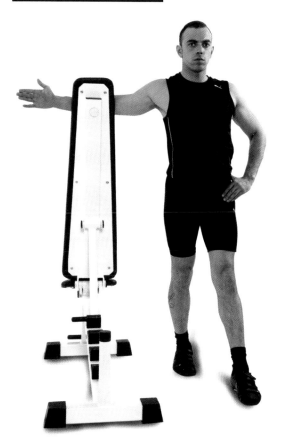

ADVANCED VERSION: STRETCHING THE WHOLE CHEST AT ONCE

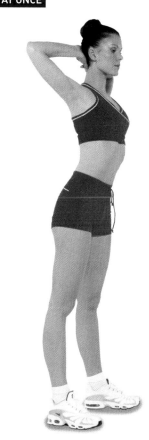

Stand with one leg in front of the other, torso straight, and one hand on your waist. Lift your other arm to shoulder level and push the inside part of your forearm against the support. To intensify the stretch in the chest muscles, gently push your arm against the support. Hold this position for 20 to 30 seconds while breathing slowly, and then repeat the same exercise on the other side.

Stand with your legs slightly apart, feet parallel, buttocks and abdominal muscles contracted, and hands behind your head with fingers intertwined. Spread your elbows toward the outside to stretch your chest muscles and shoulders. Hold the stretch for 20 to 30 seconds while you breathe slowly, then relax gently. This exercise stretches your chest muscles and shoulders while opening your rib cage.

STRETCHES FOR THE ARMS AND FOREARMS

The muscles in the arms are some of the most frequently used in the body, so it is a good idea to tone them using specific stretches. In addition, stretching will help prevent pain in the elbow and wrist joints, which is relatively common.

BICEPS AND CHEST

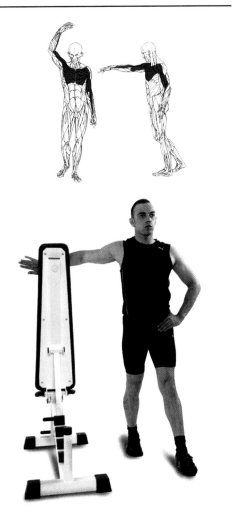

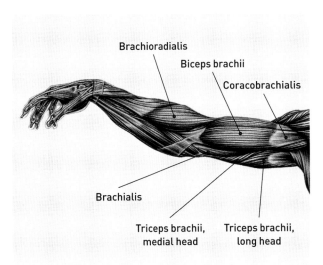

Brachioradialis
Biceps brachii
Coracobrachialis
Brachialis
Triceps brachii, medial head
Triceps brachii, long head

This exercise stretches the biceps and chest muscles.
Stand next to a support with one leg in front of the other, torso straight, and left hand on your waist. Put your right arm out straight at shoulder height and press the outer part of your forearm against the support. To increase the stretch in your chest muscles, push your arm gently against the support. Hold the stretch for 30 seconds while breathing slowly and regularly, then relax. Repeat the stretch on the other side.

ADVANCED VERSION

ADVANCED VERSION WITH HAND ROTATION

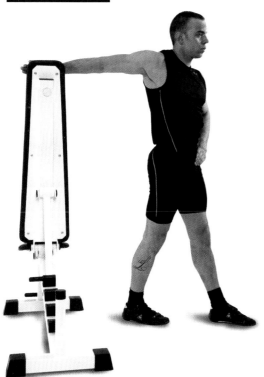

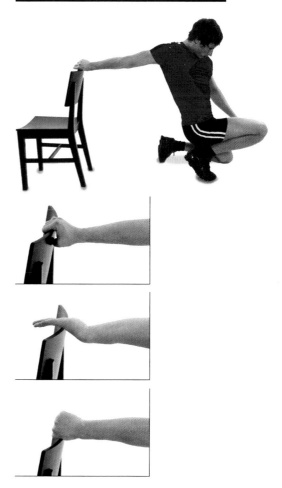

Stand with your back to a support and one leg in front of the other. Put one hand on your waist. Stretch the other arm behind you at shoulder height and place the back of the hand against the support. Hold the stretch for 30 to 40 seconds while breathing slowly, then relax. Repeat on the other side.

Crouch down next to a chair and place one hand on the chair back. Pivot very slowly so that you turn your back to the chair. Rotate your wrist from high to low and from low to high to really stretch the heads of the biceps muscle. Do not make any jerky movements, because your muscle is in a vulnerable position. Breathe slowly and regularly throughout the stretch. This exercise stretches the biceps very well.

TRICEPS

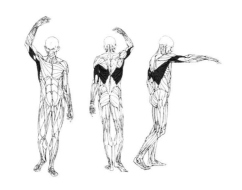

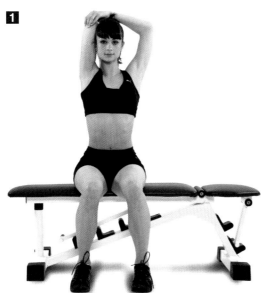

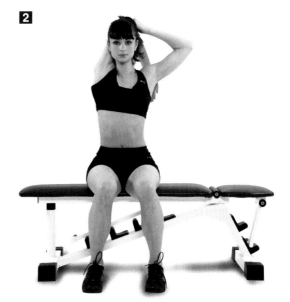

This exercise stretches the triceps.

Sit on a bench with your feet flat on the floor for stability. Bend your right arm behind your head and grab your right elbow with your left hand. Pull gently **1**. Keep pulling on your elbow to intensify the stretch **2**. When you have reached the desired position, hold it for 30 to 40 seconds while breathing slowly, deeply, and regularly. Repeat the exercise on the left side.

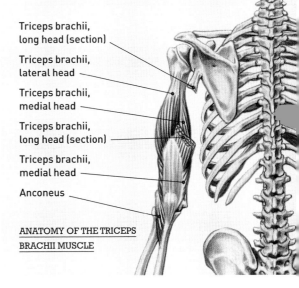

Triceps brachii, long head (section)

Triceps brachii, lateral head

Triceps brachii, medial head

Triceps brachii, long head (section)

Triceps brachii, medial head

Anconeus

ANATOMY OF THE TRICEPS BRACHII MUSCLE

VERSION WITH HAND ON THE WRIST

Sit on a bench with your feet flat on the floor for stability. Bend your right arm behind your head and put your left hand on your right wrist. Gently pull straight down. Hold this position for 30 seconds while accentuating the stretch little by little. Breathe slowly and regularly. Repeat the exercise on the left side.

STANDING VERSION

1 Stand up with your back very straight. Lift one arm up to your ear and bend it 90 degrees above your head. Grab your elbow with the other hand and pull gently while trying to bring the stretched arm behind your head. Hold the stretch for about 30 seconds while breathing slowly.

2 To intensify the stretch in your back, bend your elbow and grasp your wrist with the opposite hand. Pull gently without forcing it.

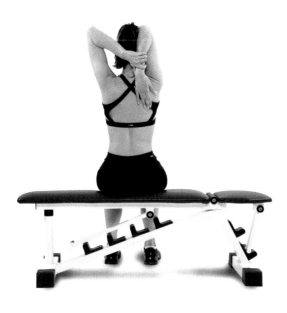

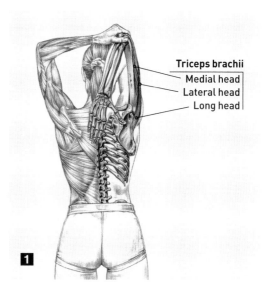

Triceps brachii
- Medial head
- Lateral head
- Long head

1

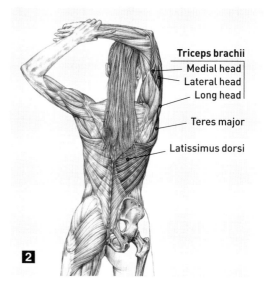

Triceps brachii
- Medial head
- Lateral head
- Long head

Teres major

Latissimus dorsi

2

WRIST FLEXORS

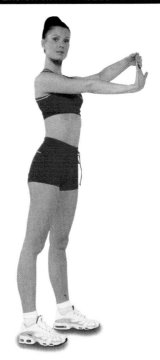

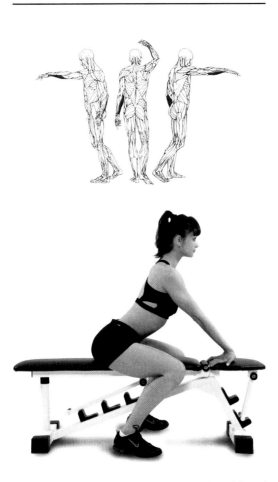

This exercise stretches the underside of the forearm (wrist flexor muscles).
Straddle a bench. Lean your torso slightly forward and keep your feet flat on the floor. Try to put the entire palm of each hand on the bench with your fingers pointing back toward you. Hold the position for 30 seconds while breathing slowly.

Stand up with your feet slightly apart and torso very straight. Straighten one arm in front of you at shoulder height with your hand extended and fingers pointing up. With the other hand, grasp your fingers and pull gently toward you without bending your elbow to stretch the entire inside of the forearm. Hold the stretch for 15 to 20 seconds while you inhale and exhale slowly. Repeat the stretch on the other wrist. This stretches the forearms and the wrists.

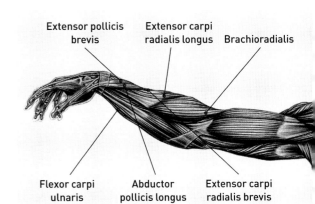

Extensor pollicis brevis — Extensor carpi radialis longus — Brachioradialis — Flexor carpi ulnaris — Abductor pollicis longus — Extensor carpi radialis brevis

STANDING VERSION WITH FINGERS POINTING TO THE SIDE

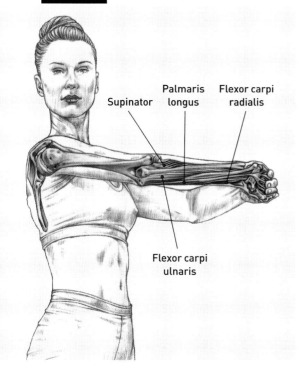

Supinator

Palmaris longus

Flexor carpi radialis

Flexor carpi ulnaris

Put one arm out in front of you at shoulder height with your wrist bent and palm facing away from you. Your fingers should be pointing to the side. With your other hand, grab your hand and pull gently so that you bring the back of your hand toward you while pushing the palm away from you. Hold this position for 30 seconds while breathing slowly and regularly. Repeat the exercise on the other wrist so you stretch the muscles in your forearm.

VERSION WITH PRAYER HANDS ▶

Stand up with your legs slightly apart so that you are in a stable position. Put your palms together at chest level with your fingers pointing up so that you stretch your flexor muscles. Hold the stretch for 30 seconds while breathing slowly and regularly.

VERSION ON YOUR KNEES

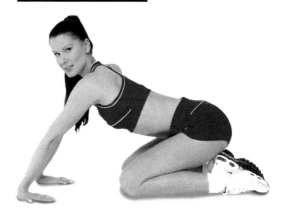

Kneel on the floor with your legs close together and your buttocks resting on your heels. Bend your torso forward and rest the palms of your hands on the floor with your fingers pointing back toward your knees. Inhale and contract your abdominal muscles while pressing on your palms. Hold this position for 20 to 30 seconds while breathing slowly and regularly, and then relax. This exercise stretches the forearms and the wrists.

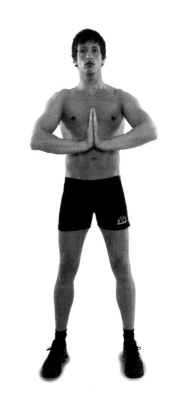

WRIST EXTENSORS

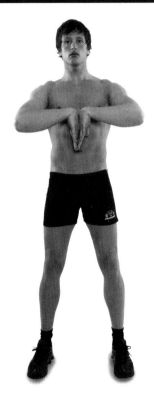

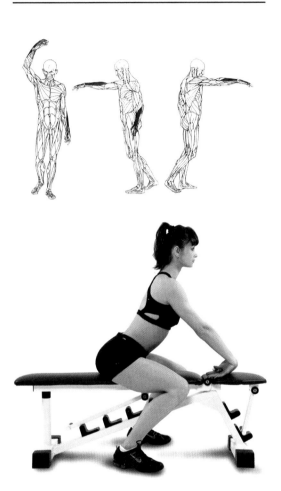

This exercise stretches the top of the forearm (wrist extensors).
Straddle a bench. Lean your torso forward and keep your feet flat on the floor. Put the backs of your hands on the bench with your fingers pointing back at your body, and try to slowly flatten your hands on the bench. Maintain the stretch for 30 seconds while breathing slowly and regularly.

Stand up with your legs shoulder-width apart for stability. Put your hands together at chest height with your fingers pointing down so that you stretch your extensor muscles. Hold the stretch for 30 seconds while breathing slowly and regularly.

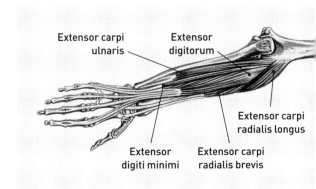

Extensor carpi ulnaris

Extensor digitorum

Extensor carpi radialis longus

Extensor digiti minimi

Extensor carpi radialis brevis

STANDING VERSION WITH FINGERS POINTING TO THE SIDE

Straighten your arm in front of you at shoulder height with your wrist bent and your palm facing you. Grab your palm with the other hand and pull gently to bring the palm toward the inside of your forearm without bending your elbow. Hold the stretch for 15 to 20 seconds while breathing slowly and regularly. Repeat the stretch on the other wrist. This exercise stretches the extensor muscles in the wrist.

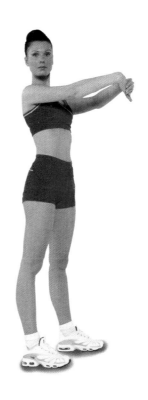

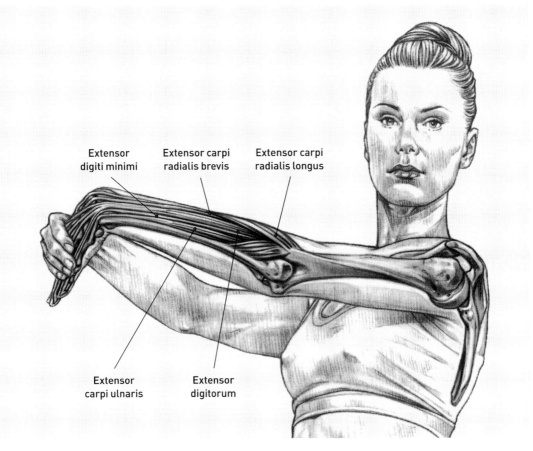

Extensor digiti minimi

Extensor carpi radialis brevis

Extensor carpi radialis longus

Extensor carpi ulnaris

Extensor digitorum

STRETCHES FOR THE LATERAL FLEXOR MUSCLES IN THE TORSO

The muscles that provide for lateral movement are very important in daily life. In addition to lateral movement, the flexor muscles in the torso support the spine, especially the lumbar spine. So these muscles help to protect the vulnerable lumbar region, which can develop pain and muscle spasms so quickly.

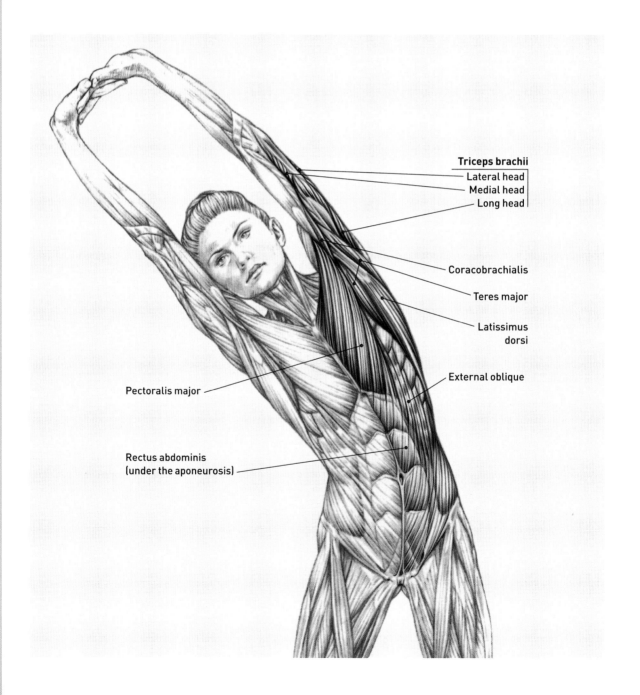

Triceps brachii
Lateral head
Medial head
Long head

Coracobrachialis

Teres major

Latissimus dorsi

External oblique

Pectoralis major

Rectus abdominis
(under the aponeurosis)

LATERAL FLEXOR MUSCLES IN THE TORSO

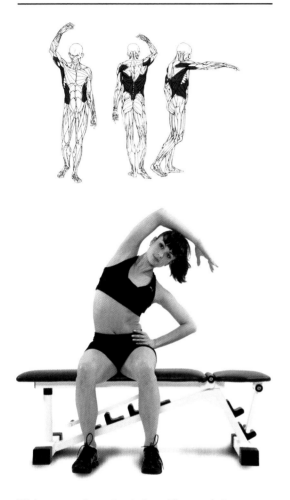

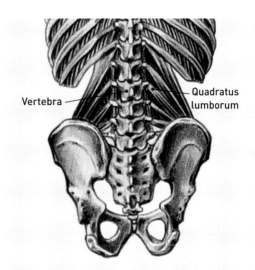

Vertebra

Quadratus lumborum

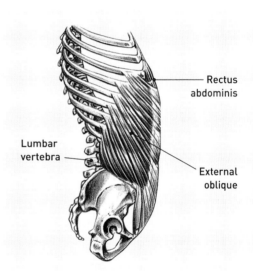

Rectus abdominis

Lumbar vertebra

External oblique

This exercise stretches the waist.

Sit down with your torso straight and put your left hand on your waist. Slightly contract your buttocks to disassociate your upper and lower body. Bend your right arm and place it above your head. Bend your torso slightly to the left to stretch your shoulder and waist thoroughly. Hold the stretch for 20 seconds, being careful to inhale and exhale regularly. Repeat the stretch on the other side.

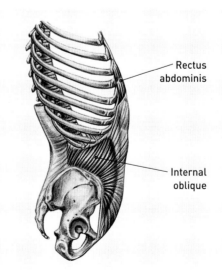

Rectus abdominis

Internal oblique

LATERAL FLEXOR MUSCLES IN THE TORSO AND BACK

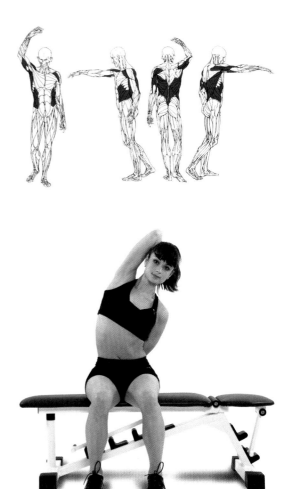

This exercise stretches the waist and back.

Sit on a bench with your back very straight. Bend your legs and put your feet flat on the floor. Stretch both of your arms above your head, intertwine your fingers, and lean slightly to the left to stretch your whole back part as well as your waist. Hold the stretch for 30 seconds while breathing regularly, then repeat the stretch leaning to the right side.

Sit on a bench with your torso straight and your feet flat on the floor. Clasp your hands behind your back with one arm going over your shoulder and the other behind your waist and then lean your torso to the side. Focus on holding your biceps against your ear so that you do not pull on your deltoid. Inhale and exhale regularly throughout the stretch. Hold this stretch for about 30 seconds, then change sides. This advanced version allows you to stretch your shoulders as well as your waist and back.

VERSION USING A STABILITY BALL

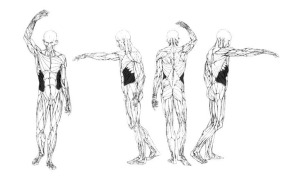

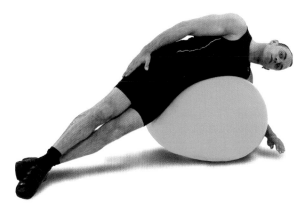

Lie on your side on a stability ball with your legs straight out away from your body. Put one hand on the floor to stabilize yourself. Keep your other arm along your body and maintain this position for about 30 seconds while inhaling and exhaling regularly. Repeat the stretch on the other side.

ADVANCED VERSION USING A STABILITY BALL

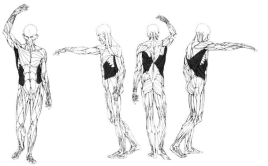

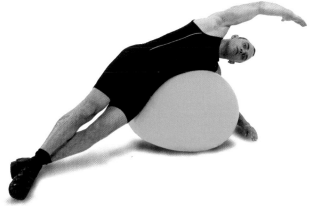

Lie on your side on a stability ball with your legs straight out away from your body. Put one hand on the floor to stabilize yourself. Hold your other arm above your head and maintain this position for 30 seconds while inhaling and exhaling slowly and regularly. Repeat this stretch on the other side. This advanced version accentuates the stretch in the obliques and the quadratus lumborum.

STANDING VERSION WITH STRAIGHT ARM

BILATERAL STANDING VERSION

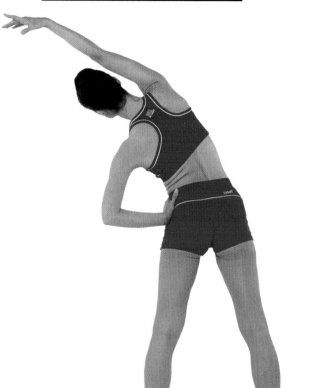

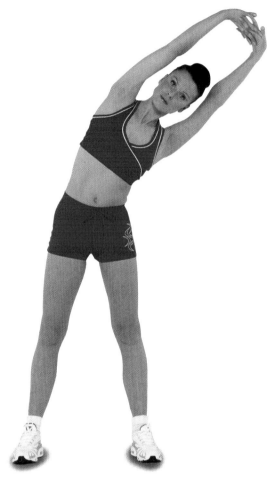

Stand with your legs apart and put your left hand on your waist and your right arm up in the air. Lean your torso to one side and then the other. Each time, hold the position for 15 to 20 seconds, breathing slowly and regularly. Repeat the stretch by changing your arm positions.

Stand with your legs slightly apart and feet pointed slightly outward to better contract your buttocks. Stretch your arms above your head and interlace the fingers. Lean your torso to the side to get an optimal stretch in the waist. Hold the stretch for 15 to 20 seconds, then come back up to your starting position. Then lean to the other side. In addition to the waist and back, this version increases flexibility in the flexor muscles of the forearms.

STRETCHES FOR THE ROTATOR MUSCLES IN THE TORSO

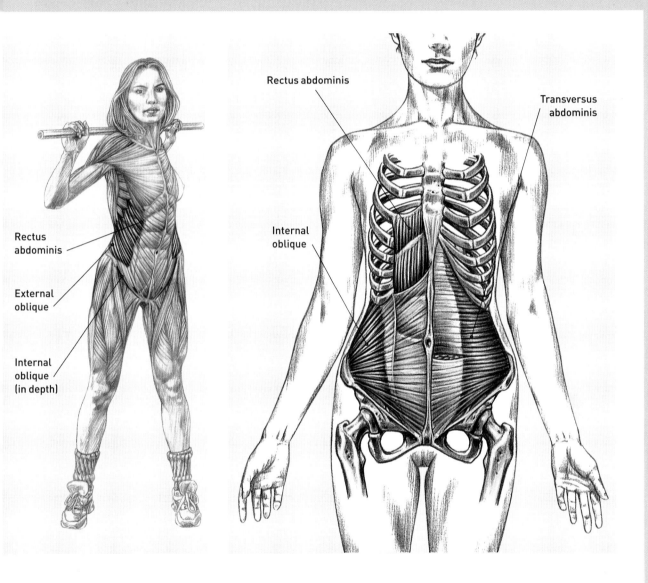

Rectus abdominis

Transversus abdominis

Rectus abdominis

External oblique

Internal oblique (in depth)

Internal oblique

In daily life, the muscles responsible for torso rotation are certainly useful but not as much as those responsible for lateral flexion. Stretching them is not a priority for sedentary people. However, for most athletes, these rotator muscles are particularly important for performance and for protecting the lumbar region. In this case, it is essential to stretch these muscles conscientiously. A good stretching program has two important roles:

→ Guarantees an optimal range of movement

→ Helps you to reestablish symmetry in your muscles

In fact, very often, only one side of the body (often the same side) is responsible for torso rotation. For example, in golf, the swing sends the ball exclusively to the left. You do not waste time swinging to the other side to send the ball to the right. This creates an imbalance in the muscular chains that can result in aches and pains or injury. A stretching program can help prevent this pitfall.

Importance of Torso Rotation for Performance

There are numerous sports in which movements are initiated by torso rotation. For example, in golf, the power of a swing comes from the back swing, during which the golfer raises the club as high as possible before bringing it down to strike the ball. For a boxer, the punch is initiated by a similar backward rotation in the trunk. It is therefore important to tone the muscles responsible for this rotation in order to

→ gain strength;
→ strengthen the muscle chains to prevent injuries, which are very common in this relatively fragile region; and
→ protect the back, particularly the lumbar region.

SEATED STRETCH FOR THE ROTATOR MUSCLES IN THE TORSO

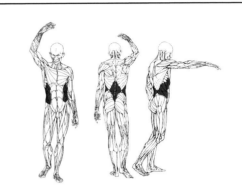

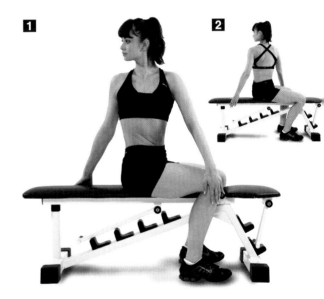

This exercise stretches the waist and lower back.
Straddle a bench with your legs bent at 90 degrees and your feet flat on the floor. Put one hand on your knee, and twist slightly so you can place the other hand behind your buttocks on the other side of the bench. Your head and your gaze are directed behind you **1**. Hold the position for about 20 seconds to create a stretch in the waist and lower back. Repeat the stretch on the other side **2**.

| ROTATOR MUSCLES IN THE TORSO, LOWER BACK, AND HAMSTRINGS | ROTATOR MUSCLES IN THE TORSO, LOWER BACK, HAMSTRINGS, AND BUTTOCKS |

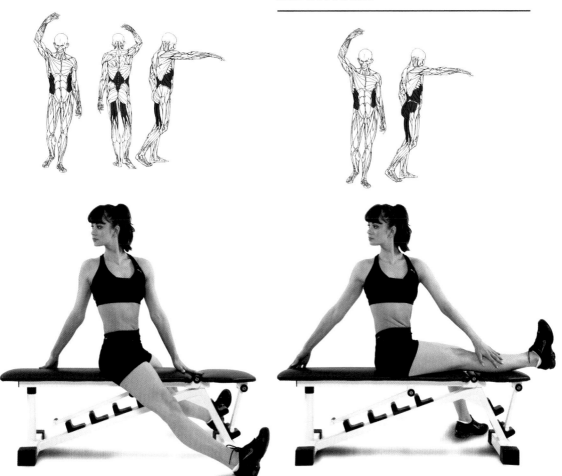

This exercise stretches the waist, lower back, and hamstrings.
Straddle a bench with your legs straight and your heels resting on the floor. Put one hand in front of you on the bench, and twist slowly so you can put the other hand behind your buttocks on the side of the bench. Hold for about 30 seconds to create a stretch in the waist, the lower back, and the back of the thighs. Then repeat the stretch on the other side.

This exercise stretches the waist and lower back as well as the hamstrings and buttocks.
Straddle a bench and stretch your right leg out in front of you. The other leg should stay bent at a right angle with your foot planted firmly on the floor. Twist your torso to the right and put your left hand on your right knee. Put your other arm behind you on the bench in line with your body. Your head and your gaze are directed behind you. Hold the stretch for 30 seconds, being careful to breathe regularly. Repeat the exercise on the other side.

ADVANCED VERSION

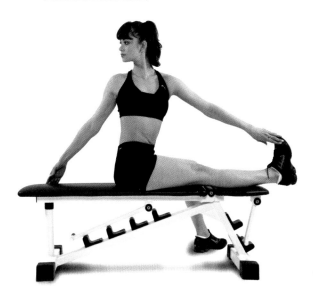

Use the same position as in the previous exercise, but grab the tip of your right foot with the left hand instead of putting your hand on your knee. This will increase your rotation.

LYING STRETCH FOR THE ROTATOR MUSCLES IN THE TORSO

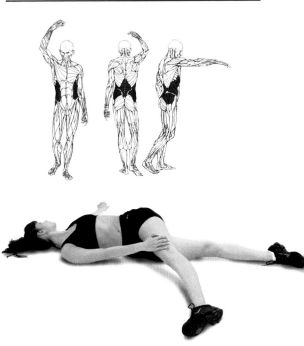

This exercise stretches the rotator muscles in the torso as well as the hips. Lie on your back with your head turned to the left and your shoulders pressed into the floor. Straighten your right leg in line with your body and put your left arm out to the side, perpendicular to your body. Pivot your pelvis to bring your left leg over your right (keeping the leg straight) until your foot is resting on the floor. Hold your left leg with your right hand and maintain the stretch for 20 seconds while breathing slowly and regularly. Then repeat the exercise on the other side.

ADVANCED VERSION

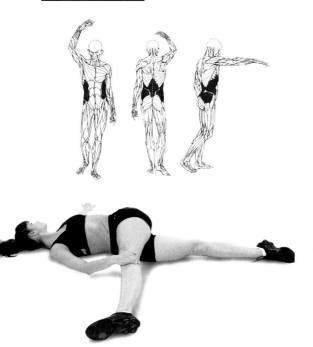

VERY ADVANCED VERSION

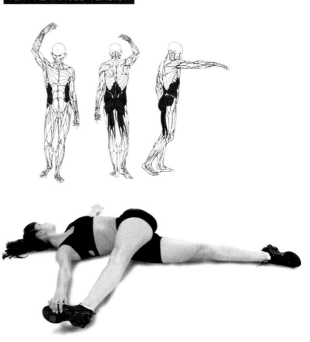

Lie on your back with your head turned to the left and your shoulders pressed against the floor. Straighten your right leg in line with your body and put your left hand out to the side, perpendicular to your body. Pivot your pelvis and put your left leg over your right (keeping the leg straight) until it forms a right angle with the other leg and the side of your foot rests on the floor. Hold it with your right hand and maintain the stretch for 20 seconds while breathing slowly and regularly. Then repeat the exercise on the other side.

Lie on your back with your head turned to the left and your shoulders pressed against the floor. Straighten your right leg in line with your body and put your left hand out to the side, perpendicular to your body. Pivot your pelvis and put your left leg over your right (keeping the leg straight). Bring the leg as high as possible and grab the tip of your foot with your right hand. Hold the stretch for 15 to 20 seconds while breathing regularly. Most important, be sure to perform this stretch gently, without forcing anything.

VERSION WITH BENT LEGS

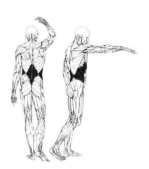

Lie on your back with your arms out to the sides and your shoulders pressed into the floor. Squeeze your legs together, bend them at a right angle, and lift them into the air. Turn your head to the left and twist your lower body to the right until your entire right leg is resting on the floor **1**. Hold this position and take the time to relax and breathe deeply. Then, repeat the exercise on the other side: legs twisted to the left while your head is turned to the right **2**.

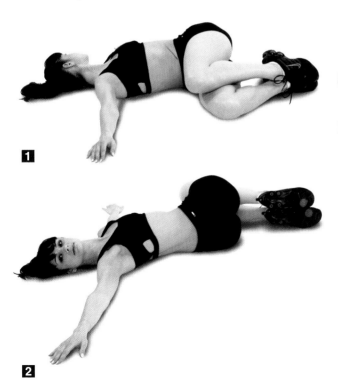

VERSION WITH STRAIGHT LEGS

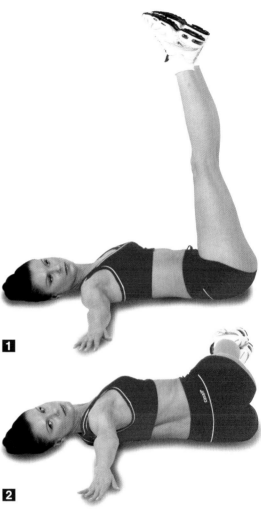

Lie on your back with your arms out to the sides and your shoulders pressed into the floor. Squeeze your legs together and hold them straight up in the air **1**. Turn your head to the right and twist your lower body to the left until your entire left leg is resting on the floor **2**. Hold this position and take the time to relax and breathe deeply. Then, repeat the stretch on the other side: straight legs squeezed together and lowered to the right while your head is turned to the left. Most important, do not force anything and be sure to breathe slowly and regularly so that your muscles can relax even more.

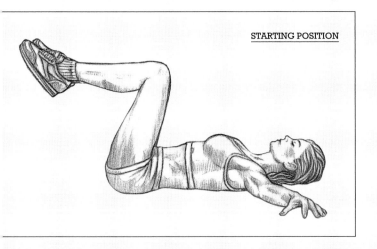

STARTING POSITION

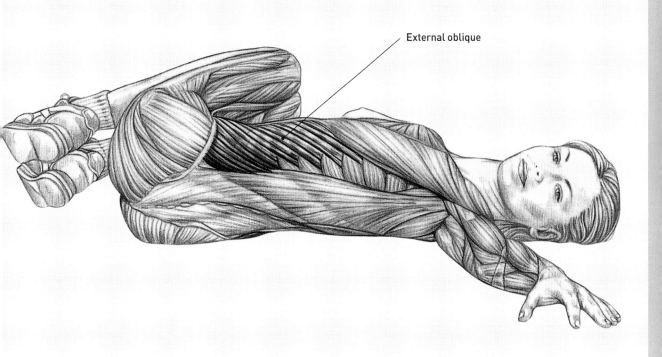

External oblique

ROTATOR MUSCLES IN THE TORSO
AND THE LOWER BACK

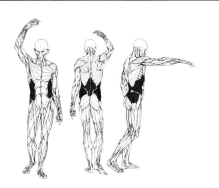

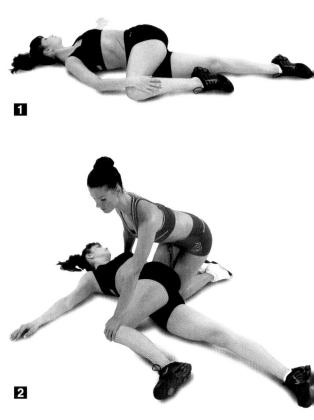

This exercise stretches the entire spinal column.

Lie on your back with your right leg stretched out in line with your body, your shoulders pressed into the floor, your arms out to the side, the palms of your hands pressed into the floor, and your head turned to the left. Bend your left leg and bring it over your right leg until it is touching the floor from the knee to the foot **1**. Breathe slowly and regularly so that you can let go and really relax your vertebrae. Hold the stretch for 20 seconds, then repeat the stretch on the other side. A partner can help you increase the intensity of the stretch a bit by using one hand to keep your shoulder pressed into the floor and putting the other hand on your knee **2**. Your partner must be careful not to apply too much pressure.

STRETCHES TO RELAX THE BACK

All physical activity involves the spinal column. The lower back (lumbar region) is the most heavily used. Because of the weight the discs have to support, the fluid enclosed in the discs is squeezed out. In fact, the discs act like sponges: When they are squeezed, fluid comes out. But this fluid is vital to the good health of the spine because it absorbs shock. Loss of fluid is the primary cause of backaches.

This explains why people are 1 to 2 centimeters (0.5 to 1 inch) shorter in the evening than in the morning. When people lie down at night, the pressure on the spine decreases and the discs fill up with fluid again.

PREVENTING LOWER BACK PAIN

Some people remain very stiff throughout the night. Not only do they sleep poorly, but the pressure on the spine does not decrease because of their overactive muscles. These people wake up feeling tired with persistent backaches. The kind of relaxation provided by stretching is therefore appropriate in this case. Stretching induces vertebral relaxation, encouraging better sleep and promoting healing in the lower back.

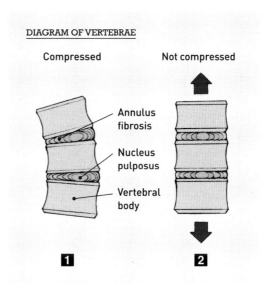

DIAGRAM OF VERTEBRAE

Compressed   Not compressed

Annulus fibrosis

Nucleus pulposus

Vertebral body

1   **2**

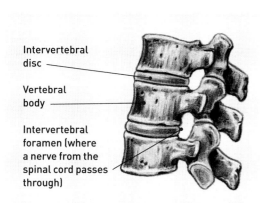

Intervertebral disc

Vertebral body

Intervertebral foramen (where a nerve from the spinal cord passes through)

1 During intense exercise, the discs can be compressed, causing the nucleus to move to the exterior.

2 When hanging from a fixed bar, the small muscles and intervertebral ligaments are stretched. The vertebrae move apart, the compression of the discs diminishes, and the nucleus pulposus is able to move back to its proper place in the center of the disc.

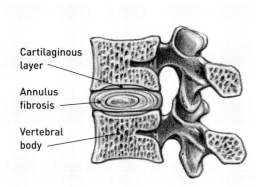

Cartilaginous layer

Annulus fibrosis

Vertebral body

RELAXING THE SPINAL COLUMN

Since the vertical position compresses the spinal column, it is imperative to stretch the back to accelerate recovery in the lumbar region. Stretching can decompress the back. The simplest stretch involves hanging from a fixed bar for at least 30 seconds. You should feel your spine lengthen freely. If, on the contrary, you feel like it is still compressed, this means your lumbar muscles are tight. You need to relax them, which is something you will learn to do over time using stretching exercises on the floor.

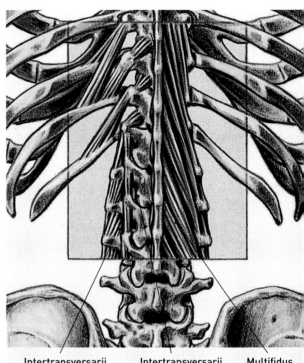

Intertransversarii lateralis   Intertransversarii medialis   Multifidus

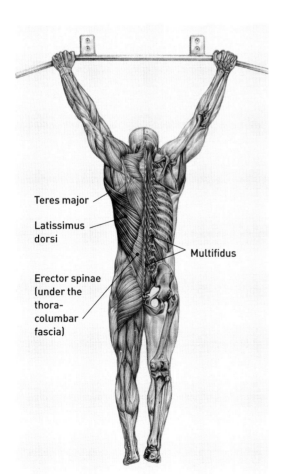

Teres major

Latissimus dorsi

Multifidus

Erector spinae (under the thoracolumbar fascia)

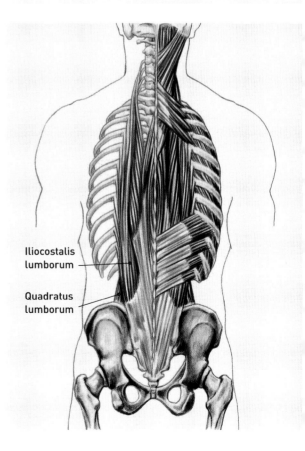

Iliocostalis lumborum

Quadratus lumborum

BACK AND ABDOMINAL MUSCLES

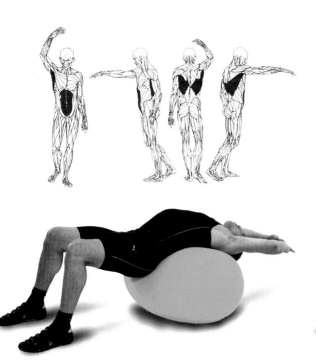

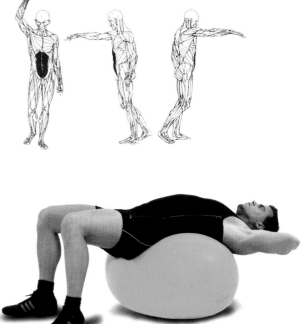

This exercise stretches the back and abdominal muscles and relaxes the spine.

Lie on your back on a stability ball with your legs bent, and plant your feet on the floor for stability. Stretch your arms over your head in line with your body. Slowly lower your buttocks toward the floor while stretching your arms as far away as possible so that you stretch your back and abdominal muscles. Hold the stretch for 30 seconds while breathing slowly and regularly.

Lie on your back on a stability ball with your legs bent, and plant your feet on the floor for stability. Bend your arms behind your neck to keep your head in line with your body. Slowly lower your buttocks toward the floor to stretch your back and abdominal muscles. Hold the stretch for 30 seconds, breathing slowly and regularly.

VERSION ON THE FLOOR

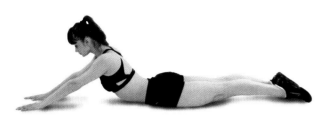

Lie on your belly with your arms out in front of you. Supporting yourself with your hands firmly on the floor, gently raise your torso. Keep your head in line with your torso and hold the stretch for 30 seconds while breathing regularly.

ADVANCED VERSION ON THE FLOOR

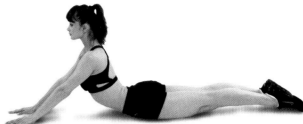

This exercise is the same as the previous one, but the stretch is more intense. Bring your hands closer to your body and raise your torso (your torso should be at approximately a 90-degree angle to your arms). This is an excellent way to stretch the abdominal muscles.

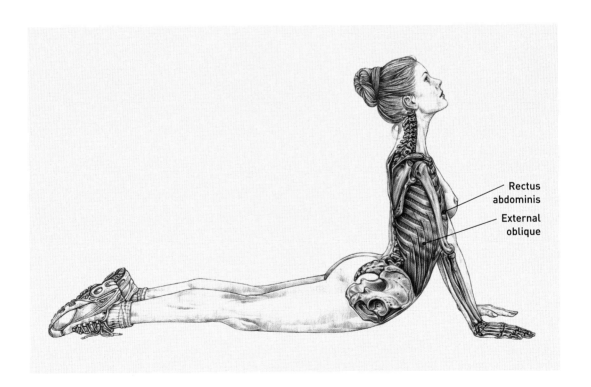

Rectus abdominis

External oblique

Do you need to stretch your abdominal muscles?

To keep your belly flat, you should not stretch the abdominal muscles very much (either in quantity or in range of motion). That being said, it is important to stretch the psoas and iliacus muscles well. You can do this by performing lunges while keeping your torso very straight.

PSOAS MUSCLES

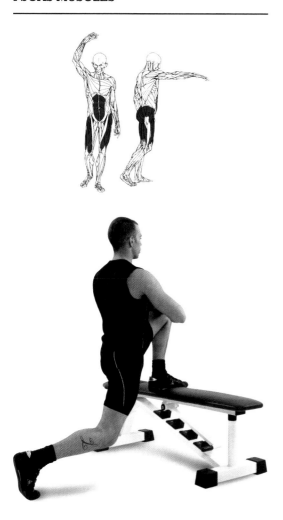

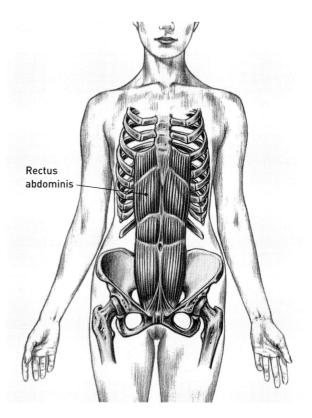

Rectus abdominis

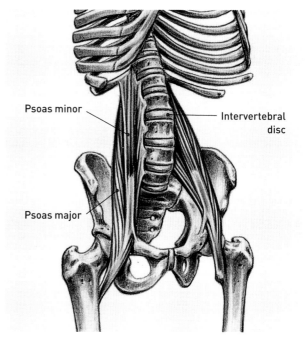

Psoas minor

Intervertebral disc

Psoas major

This exercise stretches the psoas muscles and secondarily the abdominal muscles and the quadriceps.
Stand in front of a bench and do a forward lunge with your left foot on the bench. Rest your hands on your left knee. Keep your torso very straight and lower your body by bending your left knee and raising your right heel. Hold the stretch for about 30 seconds while breathing regularly.

Abdominal-Lumbar Balance

It is important to work the abdominal muscles and the erector spinae muscles in the back equally. Underworking or overworking one of these two muscle groups can cause poor posture, which can lead to other problems.

If the lower part of the erector spinae muscles (sacrolumbar mass) is too strong and the abdominal muscles are too weak, it can lead to hyperlordosis with an abdominal ptosis **1**. You can relieve this postural problem by doing abdominal strengthening exercises. Conversely, abdominal muscles that are too strong combined with weakened erector spinae muscles, particularly in the upper back (spinalis dorsi, longissimus dorsi, iliocostalis dorsi), can lead to kyphosis (a curvature of the upper back, or hunchback) with a loss of the lumbar curve **2**. You can relieve this postural problem by doing specific exercises to strengthen the erector spinae muscles.

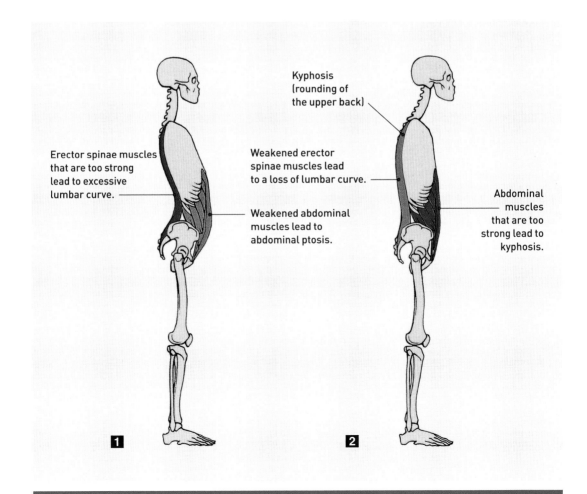

Erector spinae muscles that are too strong lead to excessive lumbar curve.

Weakened abdominal muscles lead to abdominal ptosis.

Kyphosis (rounding of the upper back)

Weakened erector spinae muscles lead to a loss of lumbar curve.

Abdominal muscles that are too strong lead to kyphosis.

1

2

LUMBAR REGION AND LATISSIMUS DORSI

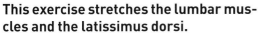

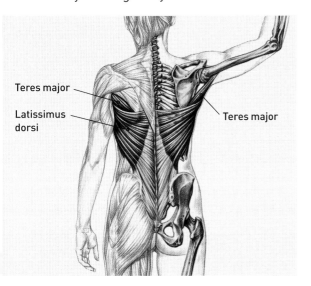

This exercise stretches the lumbar muscles and the latissimus dorsi.

Lie flat on your front on a stability ball with your knees on the floor and your arms stretched out in front of you with your hands on the floor. Hold the stretch for about 30 seconds to relax your entire back and stretch your shoulders. Breathe slowly and regularly.

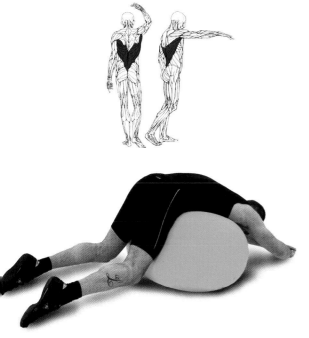

Teres major

Latissimus dorsi

Teres major

LOWER BACK AND BUTTOCKS

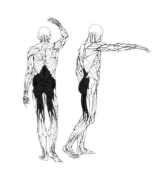

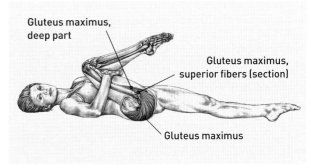

Gluteus maximus, deep part

Gluteus maximus, superior fibers (section)

Gluteus maximus

This exercise increases flexibility in the lower back and stretches the buttocks.

Lie on your back with your torso straight. One leg should be straight and the other bent. Put your hands behind the bent knee and pull gently so that you press your quadriceps against your chest. Hold the stretch for 20 to 30 seconds while you inhale and exhale slowly. Repeat the stretch with the other leg.

LATISSIMUS DORSI

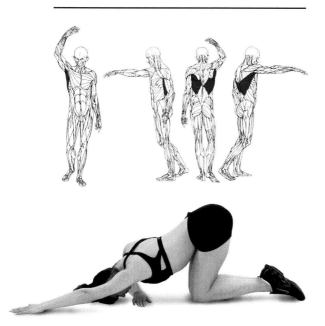

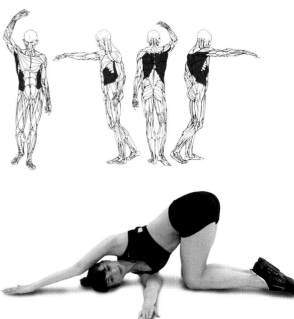

This exercise stretches the latissimus dorsi.

Kneel so that your buttocks are above your knees and your torso is leaning forward. Stretch one arm in front of you in line with your body and bend the other arm so it is perpendicular to your torso with the hand flat on the floor. Breathe regularly and hold the stretch for at least 30 seconds so that you can stretch the muscles thoroughly.

Kneel so that your buttocks are above your knees and your torso is leaning forward. Stretch one arm in front of you in line with your body and bend the other arm so it is perpendicular to your torso. Stretch it as far as possible by pivoting your torso to the inside. Breathe regularly and hold the stretch for 15 to 20 seconds. This version also stretches the rotator muscles in the torso.

STANDING VERSION

SEATED VERSION

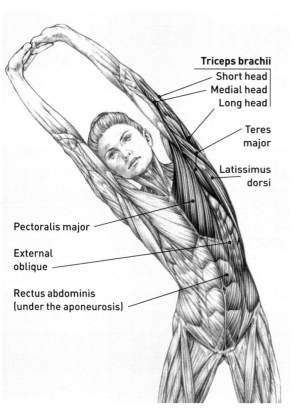

Triceps brachii
Short head
Medial head
Long head

Teres major

Latissimus dorsi

Pectoralis major

External oblique

Rectus abdominis (under the aponeurosis)

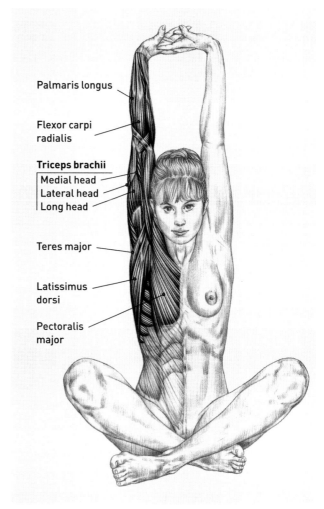

Palmaris longus

Flexor carpi radialis

Triceps brachii
Medial head
Lateral head
Long head

Teres major

Latissimus dorsi

Pectoralis major

Stand with your legs slightly apart and your arms stretched toward the ceiling. Clasp your fingers and lean to one side, keeping your head and arms in line with your torso. Hold the stretch for 30 seconds while breathing slowly and regularly. Then come back up and lean to the other side.

Sit with your legs crossed in a tailor position. Your torso should be very straight and your arms stretched up into the air. Clasp your fingers and turn your hands so that your palms are facing the ceiling. Push your hands toward the ceiling. Hold the stretch for 30 seconds while inhaling and exhaling regularly.

STANDING VERSION WITH LATERAL ROTATION

BACK, TRAPEZIUS, AND HAMSTRINGS

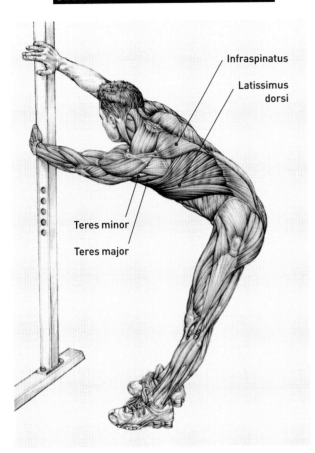

Infraspinatus

Latissimus dorsi

Teres minor

Teres major

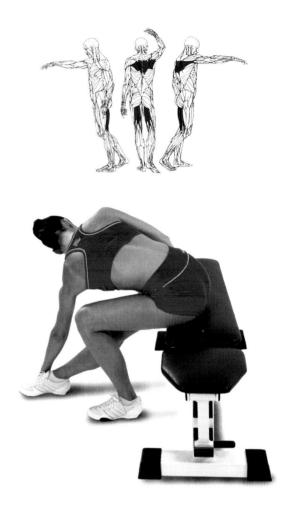

Stand with your legs slightly apart in front of a fixed vertical support. Lean your torso forward and grab the support with one hand at shoulder height. Keep the arm straight. Put the palm of your other hand higher on the support, and keep that arm straight as well. Push slowly and with increasing power while pulling with the other hand. Hold the stretch for 15 to 20 seconds while inhaling and exhaling slowly. Then relax and switch your arms.

This exercise stretches the back and trapezius muscles and increases flexibility in the hamstrings of the stretched leg.
Sit on a bench with your left leg bent and your left foot flat on the floor. Your right leg should be straight and your right foot should also be flat on the floor. Lean your torso forward and put your left hand on the outside of your straight leg while twisting slightly. Hold this position for 15 to 20 seconds to deeply stretch your entire back while you breathe slowly and regularly. Change sides.

STRETCHES FOR THE HIPS

IMPORTANCE OF HIP FLEXIBILITY

The rotator muscles in the hip play an important role in maintaining proper lumbar curve. When these muscles are not flexible enough, their tightness pulls on the lower back, causing it to lose its natural curve. This makes the lumbar discs very vulnerable to the pressure created when standing upright. This phenomenon is exacerbated in athletes when they run or even just when they walk.

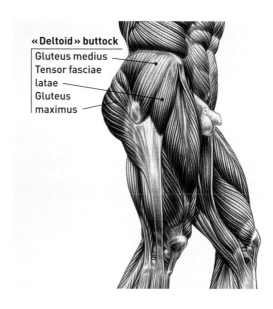

« Deltoid » buttock
Gluteus medius
Tensor fasciae latae
Gluteus maximus

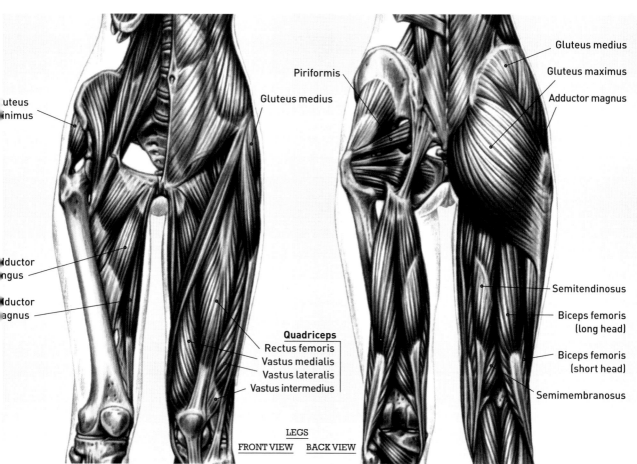

Gluteus minimus

Adductor longus

Adductor magnus

Piriformis

Gluteus medius

Gluteus medius

Gluteus maximus

Adductor magnus

Quadriceps
Rectus femoris
Vastus medialis
Vastus lateralis
Vastus intermedius

Semitendinosus

Biceps femoris (long head)

Biceps femoris (short head)

Semimembranosus

LEGS
FRONT VIEW   BACK VIEW

In sports that require hip rotation, such as golf, this stiffness interferes with proper execution of the movements. Therefore, as an athlete, you must pay special attention to the flexibility in the rotator muscles. The same is true if you wish to prevent the kind of back problems that affect a large percent of the population.

A good stretch for the rotator muscles in the hip is particularly important in sports that use the hips extensively, such as soccer, martial arts, and golf. These muscles are too often neglected.

Note
In all the exercises we describe, it is very important to work on flexibility on the left side as well as the right side. In fact, it is rare for both hips to have the same degree of flexibility naturally. The stiffest rotator will bore into the lumbar region, making it even more vulnerable to injury.

HIP STRETCH ON THE FLOOR

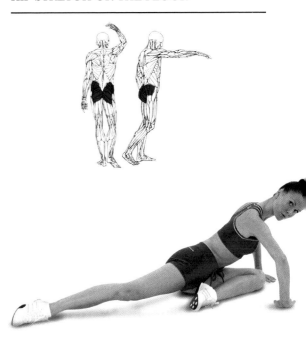

This exercise stretches the buttocks and psoas muscles.
Sit on the floor, leaning primarily on one bent leg. Stretch the other leg out in line with your body. Put your hands flat on the floor and lean your torso forward. Hold this position for about 30 seconds while inhaling and exhaling slowly and regularly. Change sides and repeat the stretch.

ADVANCED VERSION

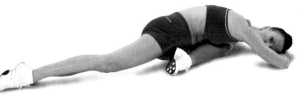

Sit on the floor, leaning primarily on one bent leg. Stretch the other leg out in line with your body. Lean your torso forward until your head is resting on your crossed forearms. Hold this position for about 30 seconds while you inhale and exhale slowly and regularly. Change sides and repeat the exercise. This stretches the buttocks, psoas, and back muscles.

HIP STRETCH ON A BENCH

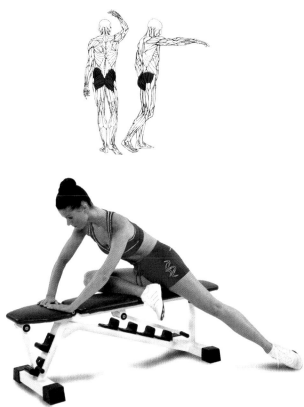

This exercise stretches the buttocks.
Put one buttock and one bent leg in front of you on a bench. Stretch the other leg behind you. Lean your torso forward and put your hands flat on the bench in front of you, keeping your arms nearly straight. Hold this position for 20 to 30 seconds, being careful to breathe regularly, before moving on to the other leg.

ADVANCED VERSION

VERY ADVANCED VERSION

FRONT VIEW

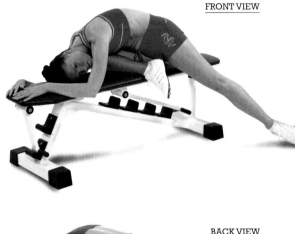

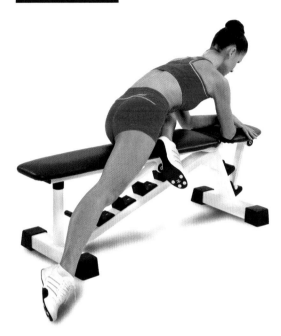

BACK VIEW

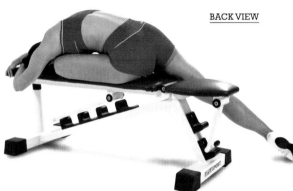

Sit on the side of a bench with your front leg bent in front of you. Stretch the other leg out behind you with the point of your foot on the floor. Bend your torso forward. Bend your arms and put your hands and forearms flat on the bench in front of you. Hold the stretch for 20 to 30 seconds while breathing slowly, then switch to the other leg. This exercise stretches the buttocks and the psoas muscles.

Sit on the side of a bench with your front leg bent in front of you. Stretch the other leg out behind you. Bend your torso forward until your head is resting on the bench with your arms bent and hands flat on the bench in front of your head. Hold the stretch for 20 to 30 seconds before moving to the other leg. This exercise stretches the buttocks and the piriformis in an even more intense fashion, and it also stretches the back.

SEATED HIP STRETCH

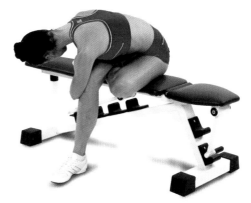

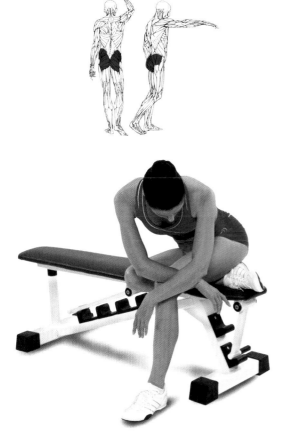

Sit on a bench with your left leg bent and tucked under your right buttock. Your right leg should be bent and your right foot should be flat on the floor. Lean forward along your right leg, tilting your head so that you really stretch the back as well as the buttocks. Hold this position for 20 to 30 seconds then switch legs.

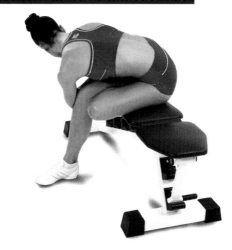

This exercise stretches the hips and buttocks.
Sit on a bench with your right leg bent and tucked under your left buttock. Your left leg should be bent and your left foot should be flat on the floor. Cross your forearms and place them on your left knee. Lean forward, keeping your head in line with your body. Hold the stretch for 20 to 30 seconds before switching to the other leg.

Sit on a bench with your left leg bent and tucked under your right buttock. Your right leg should be bent and your right foot should be flat on the floor. Lean and twist to the right. Hold this position for 20 to 30 seconds before switching to the other leg. This exercise stretches the buttocks, the back, and the waist.

FLOOR VERSION

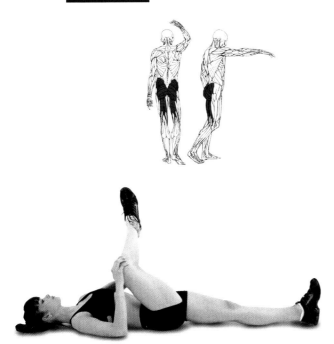

MORE INTENSE FLOOR VERSION

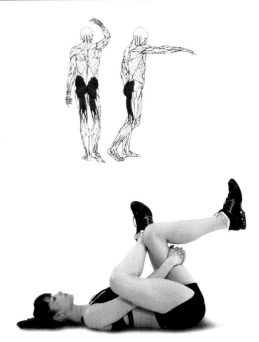

Lie on your back with one leg extended in line with your body. Bend the other leg and put it perpendicular to your body. Keep it there while holding the knee with both hands for 30 seconds. Breathe slowly and regularly. Change sides and repeat the exercise to stretch the hips and buttocks as well as the hamstrings.

Lie on your back and raise your right leg, bending it at the knee and placing it perpendicular to your body. Lift your left leg and bend it as well. Bring it toward you until the knee touches the ankle of your right leg. Grab your left thigh with both hands and hold the stretch for 30 seconds while breathing slowly and regularly. Repeat the exercise on the other side.

STRETCHES FOR THE BUTTOCKS

The buttocks are muscles that are not often used in daily life. This lack of activity explains both their lack of tone and the fact that they are often covered by a layer of unsightly fat. Stretching exercises are an excellent way to resolve this twofold problem. To obtain curved and toned buttocks, highlight the following exercises in your stretching program.

SEATED BUTTOCK STRETCH

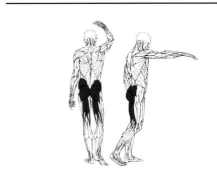

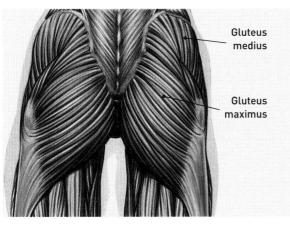

Gluteus medius

Gluteus maximus

Gluteus maximus

Gluteus medius

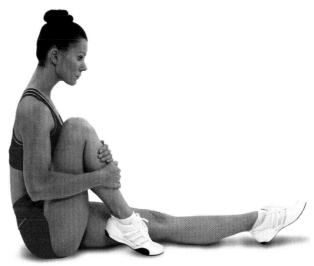

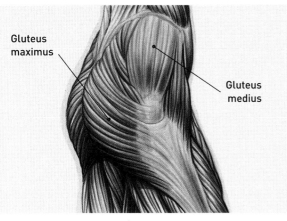

This exercise stretches the buttocks and hamstrings.

Sit on the floor with one leg stretched out in front of you. Keep the tip of your foot in line with your leg. The other leg should be bent with the toes on the floor. Put your hands on your shin and pull your leg as close as possible to your chest. Hold the stretch for 20 to 40 seconds, then change legs.

Note

There are other exercises in this book that stretch the buttocks along with the hamstrings and the adductors. You will find these stretches beginning on pages 99 and 111.

ADVANCED VERSION WITH ROTATION

Sit on the floor with your torso straight. Put your right hand behind you so that you are supported by it and your buttocks. Stretch your left leg out in front of you. Bend your right leg and put your right foot outside the left leg. Stretch your left arm out in front of you; it should go on the right side of your knee and the hand should touch your straight leg. Hold the stretch for 30 seconds while breathing regularly, then change sides. This exercise makes the buttocks and the hip rotators more flexible.

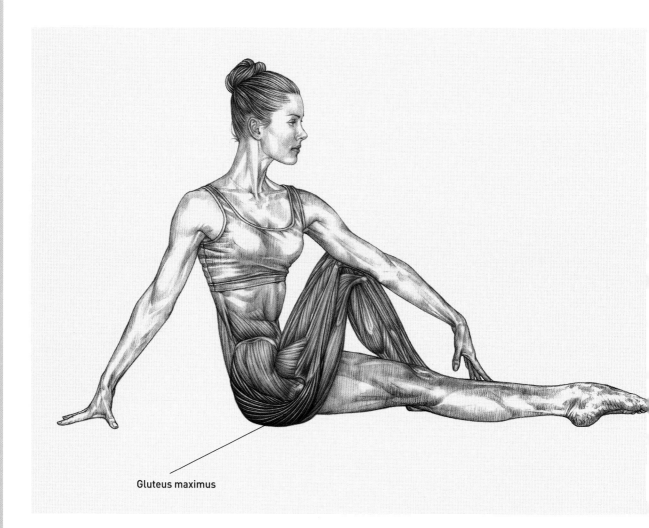

Gluteus maximus

LYING BUTTOCK STRETCH

STANDING BUTTOCK STRETCH

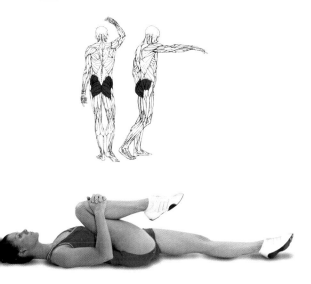

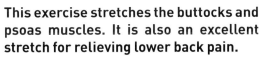

This exercise stretches the buttocks and psoas muscles. It is also an excellent stretch for relieving lower back pain.
Lie on your back with one leg bent and pulled back against your abdomen and both hands wrapped around the knee. Keeping your head in line with your body, bring your knee as close as possible to your chest. Hold this position for 30 seconds, taking the time to inhale and exhale regularly throughout the exercise. Repeat the exercise on the other side.

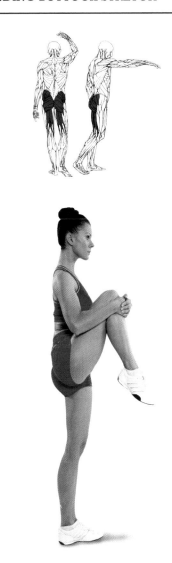

This exercise helps increase flexibility in the buttocks and hamstrings. It also improves balance, which is very important in preventing falls.
Stand with your torso very straight and lift one bent leg. Pull your knee as close as possible to your chest and keep your foot pointed in line with your leg. Wrap both hands around your knee and hold the position for 30 seconds. Breathe slowly and regularly during this stretch.

BUTTOCK STRETCH
USING A BENCH

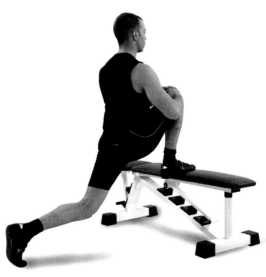

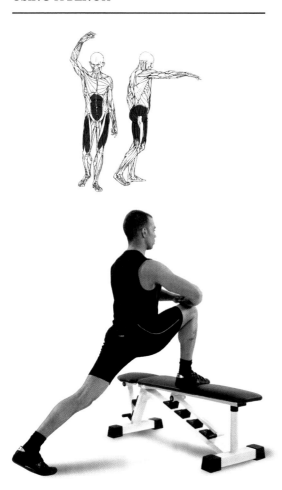

Stand in front of a bench or a step with your torso very straight. Do a forward lunge, putting your front foot on the bench. Put your hands on the front knee and lower your body by bending the front knee and lifting the heel of your back foot. Be sure to hold your torso very straight. Stay in this position for about 30 seconds and breathe regularly. Repeat the stretch on the other side. The front thigh gets more of a stretch the more you bend your back leg.

This exercise stretches the buttocks, quadriceps, hamstrings, and abdominal muscles; increases flexibility in the hip flexors; and improves balance.
Stand in front of a bench or a step and do a forward lunge, putting your front foot on the bench. The larger the lunge, the greater the stretch you will feel. Your back leg should stay very straight so that the stretch involves both thighs at the same time. Hold the stretch for 30 seconds while breathing slowly and regularly. Then change sides.

VERSION WITH BOTH FEET ON THE FLOOR

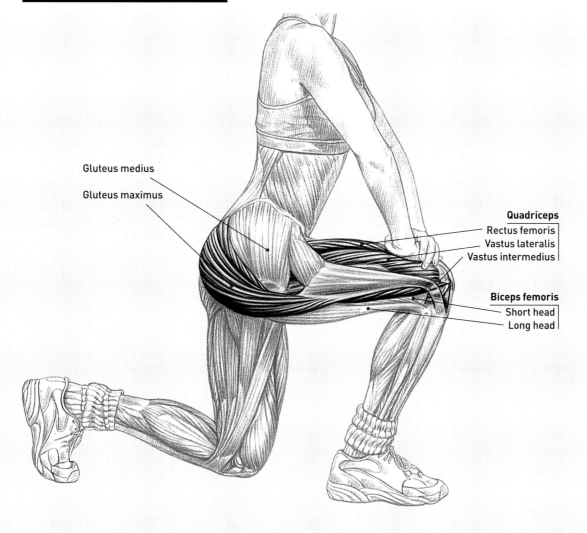

Gluteus medius

Gluteus maximus

Quadriceps
Rectus femoris
Vastus lateralis
Vastus intermedius

Biceps femoris
Short head
Long head

Put your left knee on the floor with your thigh in a vertical position. Keep your right foot flat on the floor for support. Your right thigh should be in a horizontal position. Cross your hands and place them on the right knee. Hold this position for about 30 seconds while inhaling and exhaling slowly and regularly, then switch legs.

STRETCHES FOR THE QUADRICEPS

You can have attractive thighs if you work your quadriceps regularly. Stretches will lengthen and tone your quadriceps.

Toned quadriceps muscles are required in almost all sports for good performance.

Before any exercise, it is very important to thoroughly warm up the muscles as well as the knees by stretching the thighs. After a workout, thigh stretches promote recovery and decrease muscle stiffness.

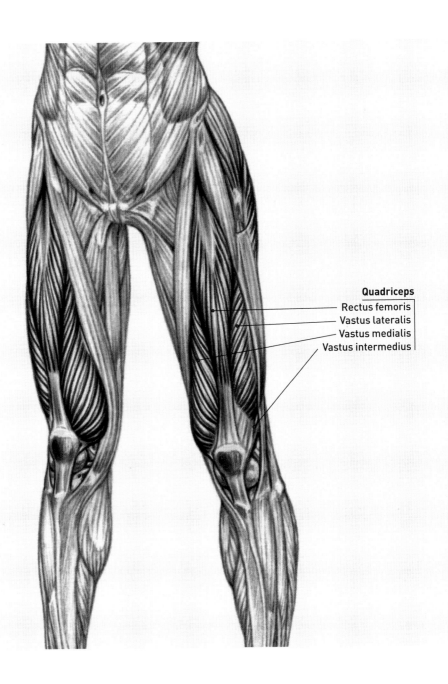

Quadriceps
Rectus femoris
Vastus lateralis
Vastus medialis
Vastus intermedius

Preventing Knee Pain

Knee problems are very common both in daily life and in sports. Some sports (such as those involving balls or rackets as well as combat sports, running, skiing, and biking) are more often associated with knee pain. Knee pain occurs so often because of two tension imbalances:

→ An imbalance between the tension exerted by the hamstrings on the menisci and the tension exerted by the quadriceps
→ An imbalance in tension between the four muscles that make up the quadriceps

These muscles naturally cannot pull with equal force on the patella, which makes the patella unstable. As a result of these imbalances, the knee joint is in a precarious position because the tension is not equal from the side or in the front.

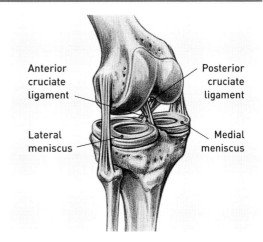

A stretching program must do the following:

→ Rebalance the tension while reducing the tension on the patella
→ Strengthen the thigh muscles so that they can protect the knee joint more effectively

A complete training program to help the knees should focus on the quadriceps and the hamstrings at the same time.

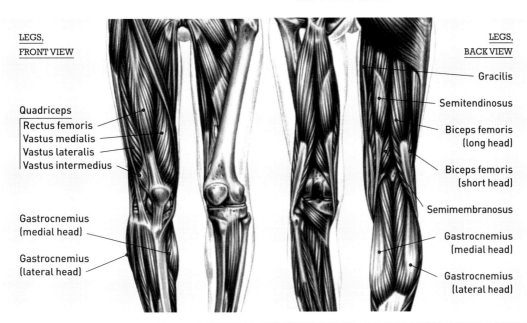

BILATERAL QUADRICEPS STRETCH

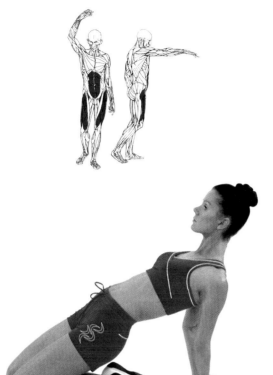

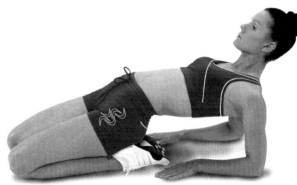

Sit on your knees and lean back. Your buttocks should rest on your heels, and your elbows should be directly under your shoulders with your forearms on the floor parallel to your body. Tightly contract your buttocks to avoid arching your lumbar spine and to stretch your quadriceps muscles. Hold the stretch for 30 seconds while inhaling and exhaling slowly and regularly.

This exercise stretches both of the quadriceps at the same time, as well as the abdominal muscles.

Sit on your knees with your buttocks resting on your heels. Place your hands flat on the floor with your fingers pointing backward. Contract your buttock muscles so that you do not curve your lumbar spine and lift your buttocks away from your heels. This will give you a good stretch in the quadriceps. Hold this position for about 30 seconds while you inhale and exhale slowly and regularly.

UNILATERAL QUADRICEPS STRETCH

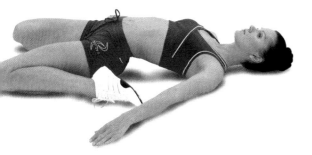

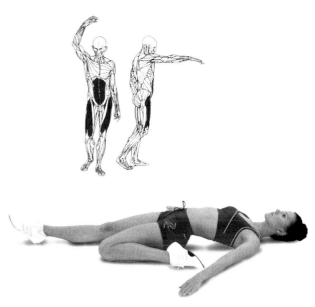

Lie on your back with your arms slightly apart and bend your legs around your body. Be careful not to arch your back too much. Your head should stay in line with your body for better oxygenation. Hold the stretch for 30 seconds while breathing slowly and regularly.

This exercise stretches the quadriceps one at a time, as well as the abdominal muscles.
Lie on your back with straight legs and arms slightly spread out. Bend one of your legs to the side and be careful not to arch your back too much. Keep your head in line with your body for better oxygenation. Hold the stretch for 30 to 50 seconds while breathing slowly and regularly. Change sides.

BALANCING QUADRICEPS STRETCH

STANDING QUADRICEPS STRETCH

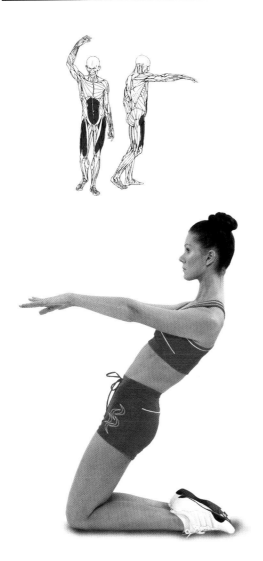

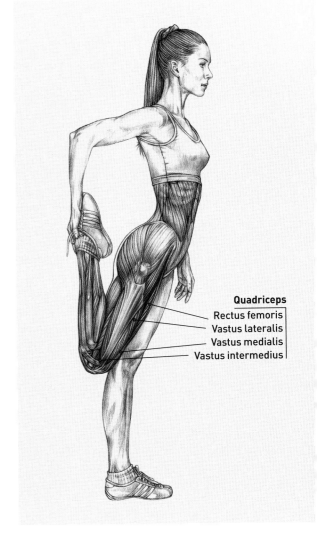

Quadriceps
Rectus femoris
Vastus lateralis
Vastus medialis
Vastus intermedius

This exercise stretches the quadriceps while also working on balance and the abdominal muscles.

Get on your knees and stretch your arms out in front of you horizontally. Lean back gently until your shoulders are above your feet. You must really contract your buttock muscles so that you do not arch your lumbar spine. Hold this position for about 30 seconds while inhaling and exhaling slowly and regularly.

This exercise stretches the quadriceps and requires balance work too.

Stand with your legs squeezed together and keep your back very straight. Bend your right leg back and grab the foot with your right hand, bringing your heel as close to your buttocks as possible. Contract your buttocks to avoid arching your lumbar spine. Hold this position for about 30 seconds while inhaling and exhaling slowly and regularly. Change sides and repeat the exercise.

ADVANCED VERSION

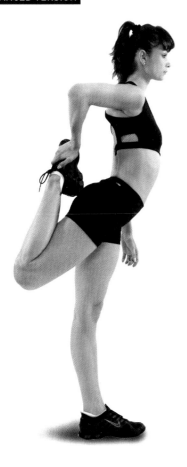

STRAIGHT TORSO VERSION USING A SUPPORT

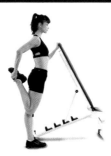

Stand with your legs squeezed together and keep your back very straight. Place your left hand at shoulder level and grab a fixed support. Bend your right leg back and grab your foot with your right hand, bringing your heel as close to your buttocks as possible. Keep your entire body very straight and contract your buttocks so that you avoid arching your lumbar spine. Hold this position for about 30 seconds while inhaling and exhaling slowly and regularly. Change sides and repeat the exercise.

HORIZONTAL TORSO VERSION USING A SUPPORT

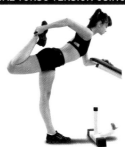

Stand with your legs squeezed together and keep your back very straight. Bend your right leg back and grab the foot with your right hand, bringing your heel as close to your buttocks as possible. Tilt your pelvis slightly so you can bring your foot above your buttocks. Keep your torso very straight and contract your buttocks and abdominal muscles so that you do not arch your lumbar spine too much. Hold this position for about 30 seconds while inhaling and exhaling slowly and regularly. Change sides and repeat the exercise. This stretch is more advanced than the previous one and requires even more balance.

Stand with your left hand at waist level holding on to a fixed support. Grab your right foot with your right hand and bring the heel close to your buttocks. Tilt your pelvis forward until the thigh is nearly horizontal. Contract your buttocks throughout the exercise. Hold this position for about 30 seconds while inhaling and exhaling slowly and regularly. Change sides and repeat the exercise. This is a more advanced stretch that also increases flexibility in the hip flexors.

BENCH VERSION

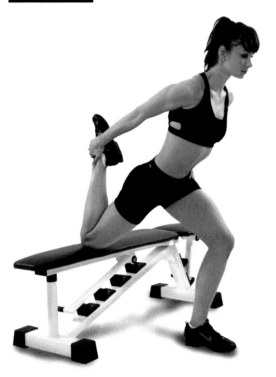

VERSION ON THE FLOOR

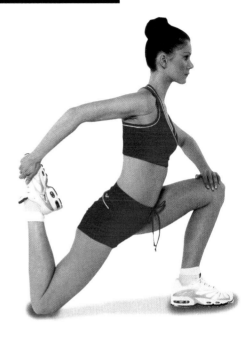

Stand in front of a bench and put your right knee behind you, resting on the bench. Grab your right foot with your right hand and keep your arm straight. Lean slightly forward and bring the heel toward your buttocks while bending your left leg. Hold this position for about 30 seconds while inhaling and exhaling regularly. Be careful not to arch your back. Change sides and repeat the exercise. This advanced stretch works on balance and coordination.

Do a forward lunge with your left leg, supporting yourself on your back knee. Put your left hand on the left knee and grab your right foot with your right hand, slowly bringing the heel toward your buttocks. Hold the stretch for a few seconds, taking the time to breathe deeply. Repeat the exercise on the other leg. This stretches the quadriceps and the adductors while improving your sense of balance.

MORE INTENSE BENCH VERSION ▶

This version is very similar to the previous version except for the position of the torso: It remains vertical and the right arm is bent. Hold this position for about 30 seconds while inhaling and exhaling regularly. Be careful not to arch your back. Change sides and repeat the exercise. This advanced stretch really requires balance.

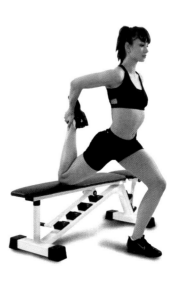

STRETCHES FOR THE HAMSTRINGS

The hamstrings, or the backs of the thighs, continue the line of the buttocks. In sedentary people, the hamstrings' chronic inactivity explains their lack of tone as well as the layer of fat often found there. In extreme cases, there can be a lot of fatty tissue called cellulite. So it is important to stretch the hamstrings in order to tone them and eliminate cellulite.

PREVENTING HAMSTRING TEARS

In athletes, hamstring tears are fairly common, especially in sports that require sprinting in an irregular fashion, such as in soccer, rugby, racket sports, ice skating, and track and field. To prevent these injuries, use gentle stretches to warm up your hamstrings well before any work involving the thighs. Stretching also increases your range of motion, which facilitates movement (especially for large strides during a sprint).

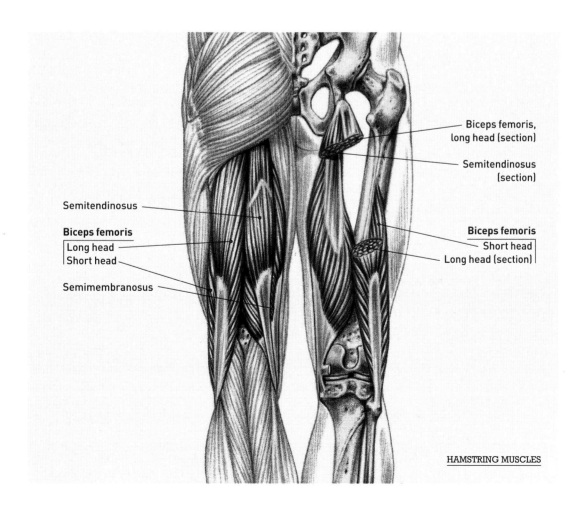

Biceps femoris, long head (section)

Semitendinosus (section)

Semitendinosus

Biceps femoris
Long head
Short head

Semimembranosus

Biceps femoris
Short head
Long head (section)

HAMSTRING MUSCLES

UNILATERAL STANDING HAMSTRING STRETCH

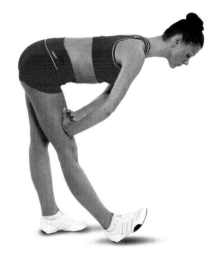

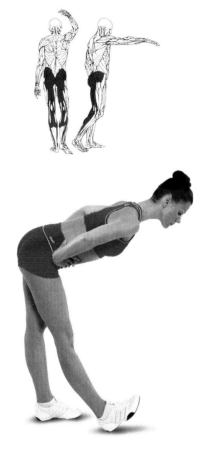

Start from a standing position and put one leg forward. Lean your torso forward and keep your head in line with your body so that you do not pull on your cervical spine. Lift the foot as much as possible, but keep the heel on the floor. To intensify the stretch, put both hands on your thigh, just above the knee. Hold the stretch for 30 to 40 seconds, and breathe slowly and regularly. Change sides and repeat the exercise. The stretch will be more intense as you lean farther forward.

This exercise stretches the hamstrings, buttocks, and calves.

Stand with your hands on your hips and put one leg forward. Lean your torso forward so it forms a right angle with the forward leg. Keep your head in line with your body so that you do not pull on your cervical spine. Lift the foot as much as possible while leaving the heel on the floor so that you also stretch the calf and work on your balance. Hold the stretch for 30 to 40 seconds while you breathe slowly and regularly. Change sides and repeat the exercise.

VERY ADVANCED VERSION

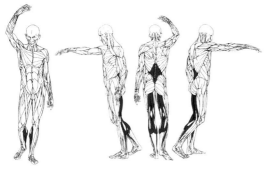

EXTREMELY ADVANCED VERSION

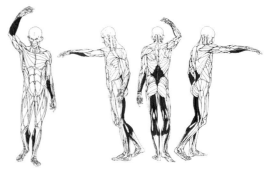

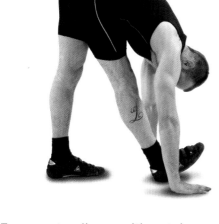

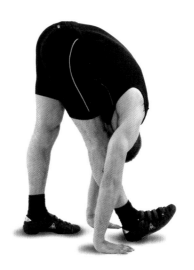

From a standing position, take one step forward. Keep the legs straight and lean your torso forward as much as possible over the front leg. Put your hands flat on the floor around the front foot. Lift the ball of the foot and leave the heel on the floor. Hold the stretch for 30 to 40 seconds while you breathe slowly and regularly. Change sides and repeat the exercise. This stretches the hamstrings, lower back, and calves.

From a standing position, take one step forward. Keep the legs straight and lean your torso forward as much as possible over the front leg. Put your hands flat on the floor as far as possible behind the foot. Lift the ball of the foot and leave the heel on the floor. Hold the stretch for 30 seconds while you breathe slowly and regularly. Change sides and repeat the exercise. This stretches the hamstrings, calves, and lower back and also increases flexibility in the wrist flexors.

BENT-LEG VERSION

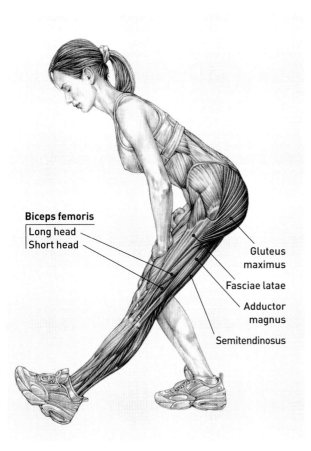

Biceps femoris
| Long head
| Short head

Gluteus
maximus

Fasciae latae

Adductor
magnus

Semitendinosus

BENCH VERSION

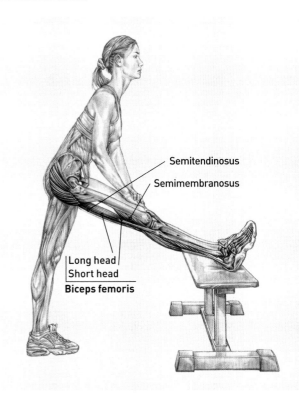

Semitendinosus

Semimembranosus

Long head |
Short head |
Biceps femoris

Stand up and take a full step forward without bending your leg. Lift the ball of the foot, but leave the heel on the floor. Lean your torso forward, keeping your head in line with your body so that you do not pull on your cervical spine. Place your hands on your thigh just above your knee. Bend your standing leg to make the hamstrings work more and involve the buttock muscle. Hold the stretch for 30 seconds while you breathe slowly and regularly. Change sides and repeat the exercise.

Stand in front of a bench. Lift your leg without bending it and place the heel on the bench. Lean your torso forward about 45 degrees, keeping your head in line with your torso. Put both hands just above the knee. Hold the stretch for 30 seconds while you breathe slowly and regularly. Change sides to repeat the exercise. This stretches the hamstrings, lower back, buttocks, and calves.

ADVANCED BENCH VERSION

Stand in front of a bench. Lift your leg without bending it, and place the heel on the bench. Lean your torso forward and put both hands on the bench next to your foot. Hold the stretch for 30 seconds while breathing slowly and regularly. Change sides and repeat the exercise. This stretches the hamstrings, buttocks, lower back, and calves.

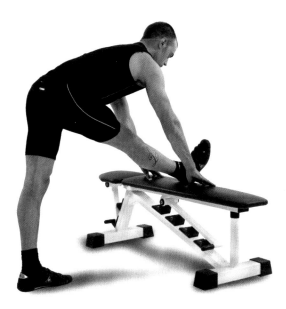

BILATERAL STANDING HAMSTRING STRETCH

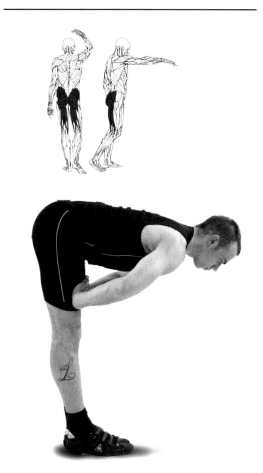

This exercise stretches the hamstrings and buttocks.
Stand with straight legs and squeeze them together. Lean your torso forward until it is at a right angle to your thighs, and then put your hands on the middle of your thighs. Keep your head in line with your torso. Hold this position for 30 to 40 seconds while inhaling and exhaling slowly.

ADVANCED VERSION

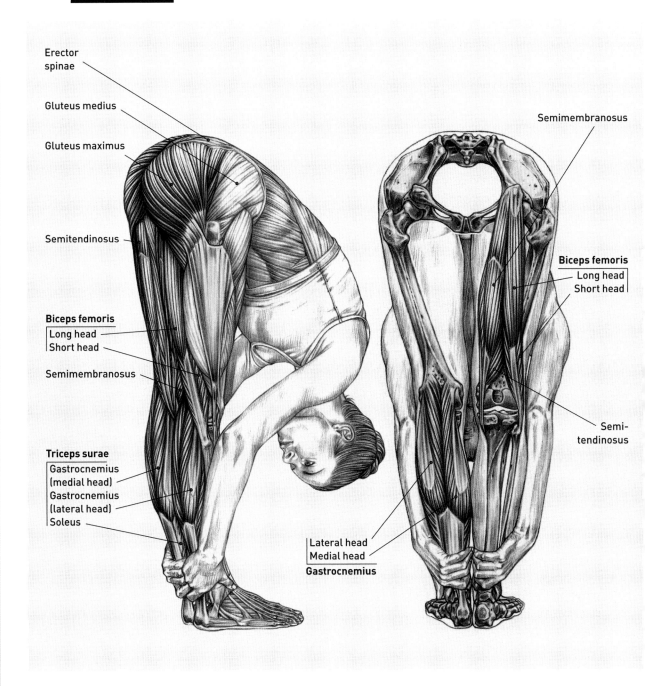

Erector spinae

Gluteus medius

Gluteus maximus

Semitendinosus

Biceps femoris
Long head
Short head

Semimembranosus

Triceps surae
Gastrocnemius (medial head)
Gastrocnemius (lateral head)
Soleus

Lateral head
Medial head
Gastrocnemius

Semimembranosus

Biceps femoris
Long head
Short head

Semi-tendinosus

Stand with your legs squeezed together and very straight. Lean your torso forward, keeping your head in line with your torso, and grab your ankles from behind. Hold the stretch for 30 to 40 seconds, breathing slowly and calmly. This exercise stretches the hamstrings and buttocks.

VERY ADVANCED VERSION

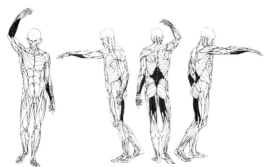

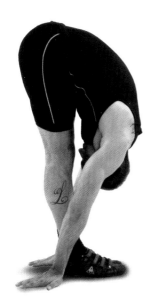

ADVANCED VERSION WITH SHOULDER STRETCH

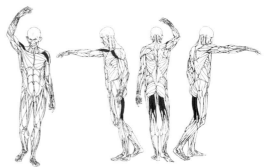

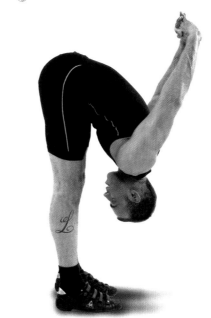

Stand with your legs squeezed together and very straight. Lean your torso forward, keeping your head in line with your torso, and place your hands flat on the floor by your heels with your fingers pointing backward. Hold the stretch for 30 to 40 seconds while breathing slowly and calmly. This exercise stretches the hamstrings and lower back. It also increases flexibility in the wrist flexor muscles.

Stand with your legs squeezed together and very straight. Put your arms behind your back and clasp your fingers together. Lean forward so that your head comes down to your knees while you push your arms as far forward as possible. Hold the stretch for 30 to 40 seconds and breathe slowly and calmly. This exercise stretches the hamstrings and deltoids.

VERSION USING A BAR

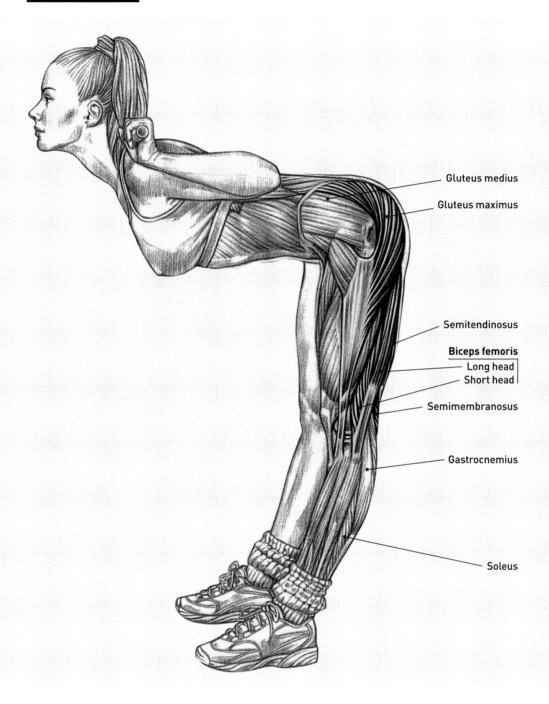

Gluteus medius

Gluteus maximus

Semitendinosus

Biceps femoris
Long head
Short head

Semimembranosus

Gastrocnemius

Soleus

Begin the movement standing with straight legs slightly apart. Hold a bar with both hands behind your head. The bar should rest on your trapezius muscles and not on your neck. Lean your torso forward to make a right angle and lift your head. Hold the stretch for 30 to 40 seconds, and inhale and exhale slowly. This exercise stretches the hamstrings, shoulders, back, and buttocks.

FLOOR VERSION

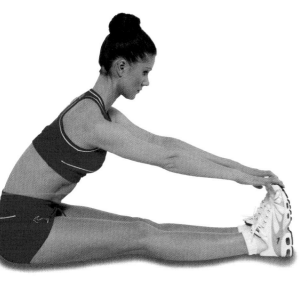

HAMSTRING STRETCH ON THE FLOOR

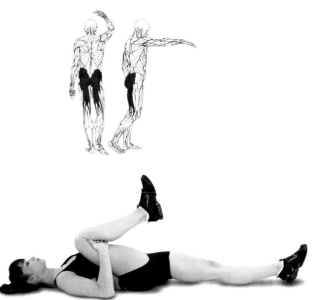

Sit on the floor with straight legs and lean your torso forward, keeping your head in line with your torso. Depending on your flexibility, grab the ends of your feet or your shins. Try to hold the stretch, and breathe slowly and regularly throughout the exercise. To relax your entire back and intensify the stretch, lean your torso forward while pulling your chest toward your thighs. If you have difficulty with this exercise, you can bend your legs slightly.

This exercise stretches the hamstrings and buttocks. It is also excellent for relaxing the spine.
Lie on your back and pull one leg back against your abdomen. Grab your thigh with both hands just under the knee. Keep your head in line with your body and bring the knee as close as possible to your chest. Hold the position for 30 seconds, taking the time to inhale and exhale regularly. Change sides and repeat the exercise.

ADVANCED VERSIONS

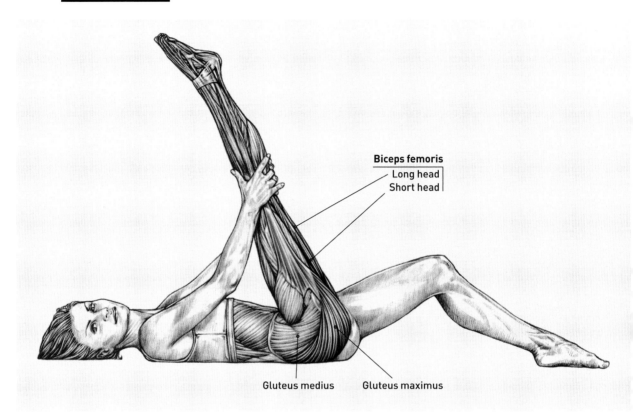

Biceps femoris
Long head
Short head

Gluteus medius   Gluteus maximus

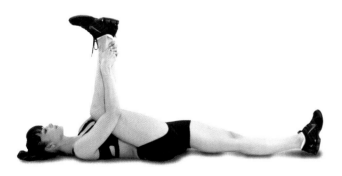

Lie on your back. Bend one leg slightly ▲ and place the foot flat on the floor. Lift the other leg, keeping it very straight, and point your foot. Grab the leg with both hands at the knee. Hold the position for 30 to 40 seconds, taking the time to inhale and exhale regularly. Repeat the exercise on the other leg to stretch the hamstrings and gluteus maximus.

▲ Lie on your back and pull one leg back against your abdomen. Grab your ankle with both hands. Keep your head in line with your body and bring the knee as close as possible to your chest with your foot straight above your knee. Hold the position for 30 seconds, taking the time to inhale and exhale regularly. Repeat the exercise on the other side to stretch the hamstrings.

VERY ADVANCED VERSION

HAMSTRING STRETCH SEATED ON A BENCH

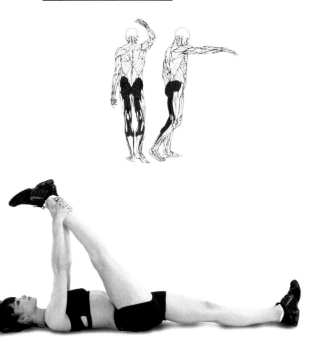

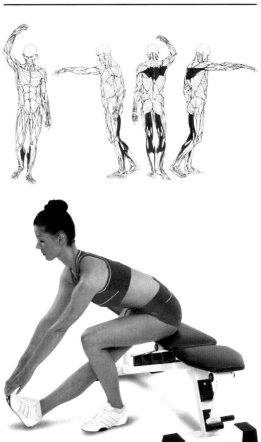

Lie on your back, and put both legs straight out in front of you. Lift one leg and grab the ankle with both hands. Your arms should be straight above your shoulders. Hold the position for 30 seconds, taking the time to inhale and exhale regularly. Repeat the exercise on the other side to stretch the hamstrings and psoas muscles.

This exercise stretches the hamstrings and increases flexibility in the calves.
Sit on a bench with one leg bent and the foot flat on the floor. The other leg should be straight, with the heel on the floor. Lean forward while keeping your back straight so that you can grab the toes of your foot with both hands. Hold the stretch for 30 seconds, and be sure to breathe normally throughout the exercise. Change sides to stretch the other leg.

TWISTING VERSION

HAMSTRINGS AND ADDUCTORS

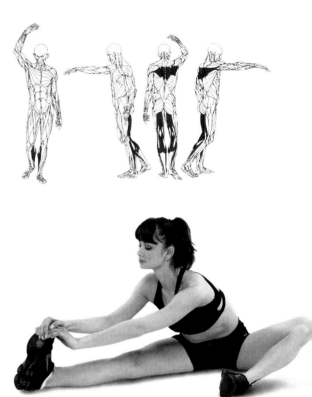

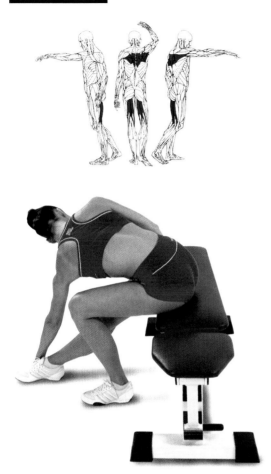

Sit on a bench with your left leg bent and your left foot flat on the floor. Your right leg should be straight and your right foot should also be flat on the floor. Lean forward and put your right hand on the bench and put your left hand on the outside of your right foot. Hold this position for 30 seconds, and be sure to breathe normally during the exercise. Change sides to stretch the other leg. Keeping the foot of the straight leg flat on the floor makes this stretch less intense because it stretches only the hamstrings.

This exercise stretches the hamstrings and, to a lesser degree, the adductors.
Sit on the floor with one leg bent and the other straight in front of you. Grab the tip of the foot of your straight leg with both hands and hold the stretch for 30 seconds, and inhale and exhale slowly and regularly. Change sides and repeat the stretch.

STRETCHES FOR THE ADDUCTORS

In daily life, the adductor muscles are not often used. Since they naturally have weak muscle tone, it is a good idea to strengthen them through regular stretching. In numerous sports—and especially in those requiring side-to-side movements, such as tennis—the adductors are heavily used. This explains why they are often the site of extremely painful injuries. Runners and athletes who play tennis or combat sports must be especially careful to increase flexibility in the adductors.

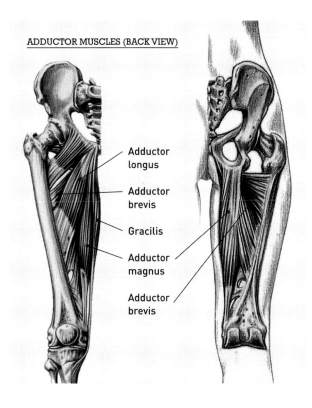

ADDUCTOR MUSCLES (BACK VIEW)

Adductor longus

Adductor brevis

Gracilis

Adductor magnus

Adductor brevis

⚠ Wide Splits: Warning!

Doing a wide split to the side or front to back is seen as a sign of flexibility. However, just because you can do the splits does not mean that you are flexible. In the same way, if you cannot do the splits, it does not mean you are inflexible. Other than being impressive, the wide split is not very useful except in certain combat sports or in dance or gymnastics where it is used in a few set figures. However, all body types are not made to do the splits (see page 112). Since the splits involve only a single joint and are not extremely useful, your stretching program should not focus solely on the splits.

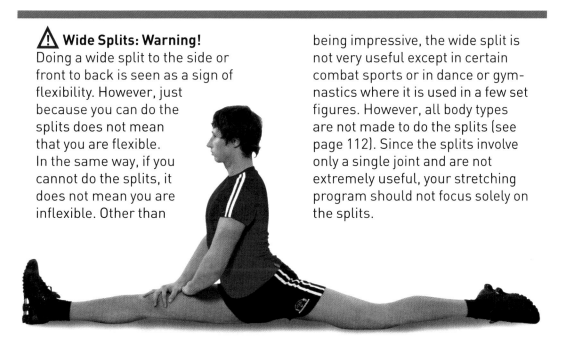

The Various Bony Morphologies of the Hip

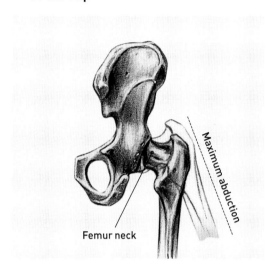

A femur neck that is nearly horizontal is called coxa vara. It limits abduction because it strikes the superior edge of the cotyloid cavity sooner.

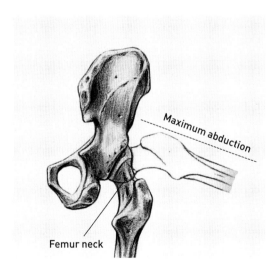

A femur neck that is nearly vertical is called coxa valga. It facilitates greater abduction.

ADDUCTOR STRETCH WITH A STRAIGHT LEG

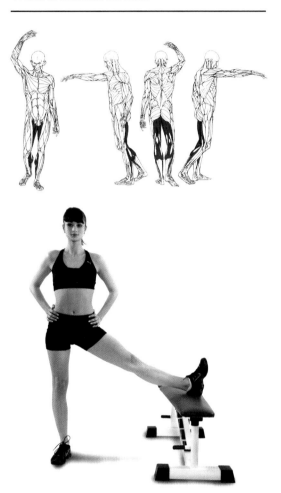

This exercise stretches the adductors, hamstrings, and calves.
Stand next to a bench with your torso and legs straight. Put both hands on your waist and put one leg on the bench supported by the heel, with the foot pointing up. Hold the stretch for 30 seconds while inhaling and exhaling slowly and regularly, then change sides. This stretch targets the adductors and hamstrings at the same time.

ADVANCED VERSION

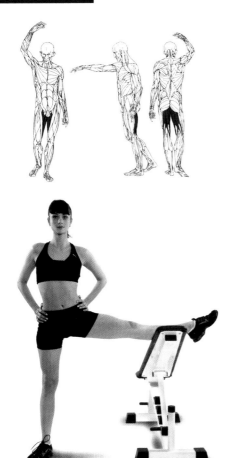

ADVANCED VERSION
WITH THE LEG TURNED IN

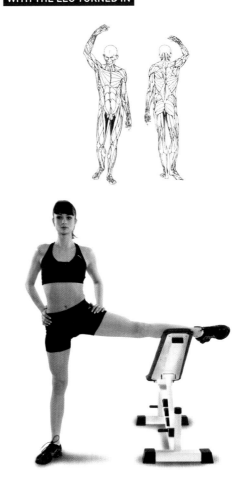

This exercise stretches the adductors and hamstrings.

Stand with your torso straight and your hands on your waist next to a support about 26 to 32 inches (65 to 80 cm) tall, depending on your height. Put one calf on the support so that your leg is straight and horizontal with your knee and foot pointing up. The foot resting on the floor should be slightly turned out. Hold the stretch for 30 seconds while inhaling and exhaling slowly and regularly, then change sides. You can also rest your thigh on the support rather than your calf to get a more direct stretch of the adductor. One advantage of that version is that you avoid twisting the knee.

This stretch is very similar to the previous one, but you should gently twist your supported leg clockwise about 45 degrees so that your knee and foot are facing front. Hold the stretch for 30 seconds while inhaling and exhaling slowly and regularly. Then change sides. This exercise stretches the adductors and the hips. Be careful not to push your knee too far.

ADDUCTOR STRETCH WITH A BENT LEG

ADVANCED VERSION

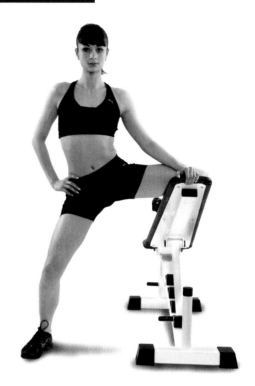

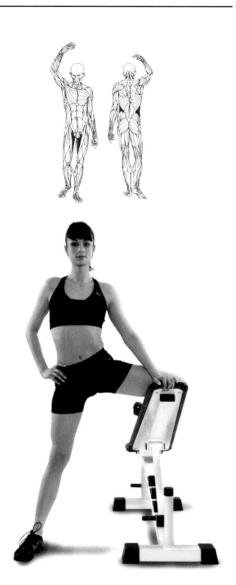

Stand near a support with your right leg slightly bent and the foot slightly pointed out. Put your right hand on your waist. Bend your left leg and rest it on the support. Put your left hand on the support and hold the stretch for 30 seconds while breathing slowly and regularly. Then change sides. By bending the leg on the floor, you increase the tension on the adductor.

This exercise stretches the adductors and hips.
Stand near a support with your right leg straight and the foot slightly pointed out. Put your right hand on your waist. Bend your left leg and rest it on the support. Put your left hand on the support and hold the stretch for 30 seconds while breathing slowly and regularly. Then change sides.

SQUATTING ADDUCTOR STRETCH

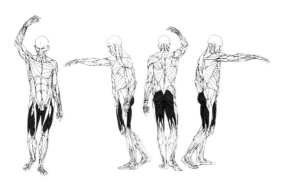

SUMO VERSION

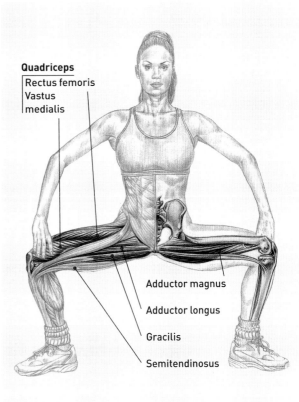

Quadriceps
Rectus femoris
Vastus
medialis

Adductor magnus

Adductor longus

Gracilis

Semitendinosus

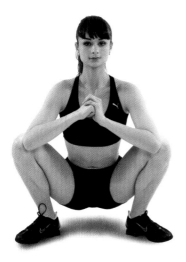

This exercise stretches the adductors, buttocks, quadriceps, and hamstrings.
Squat down with your legs apart and feet pointing out. Keep your back very straight. Put your elbows against the insides of your knees and clasp your hands. Push your knees to the outside using your elbows, but do not push too hard. Hold the stretch for 30 seconds and breathe slowly and regularly.

Begin the exercise standing with your legs apart and feet pointing out. Keep your back straight. Lower your torso until your thighs are horizontal and put your hands on your knees. Hold the position for 15 to 20 seconds, being careful to breathe normally. This exercise stretches the adductors, buttocks, and quadriceps.

SITTING ADDUCTOR STRETCH

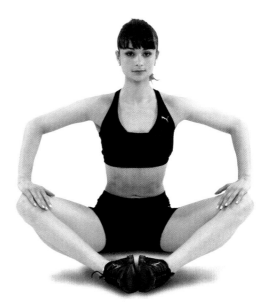

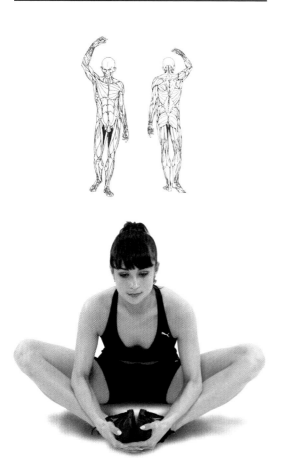

Sit in the same position as in the previous exercise, but keep your back very straight. Put your hands on your knees with your fingers pointing in and push gently to increase the stretch. Hold the stretch for 30 seconds while breathing slowly and regularly.

This exercise stretches the adductors and hips.
Sit in the tailor position with the soles of your feet touching. Lean forward slightly and grab your feet with both hands. Hold the stretch for 40 seconds, breathing slowly and regularly.

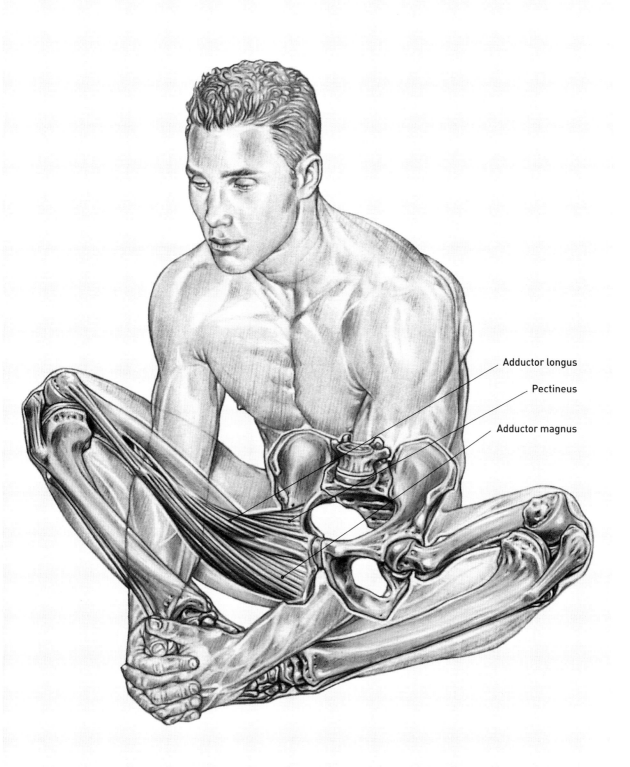

Adductor longus

Pectineus

Adductor magnus

SEATED ADDUCTOR AND HAMSTRING STRETCH

STANDING ADDUCTOR AND HAMSTRING STRETCH

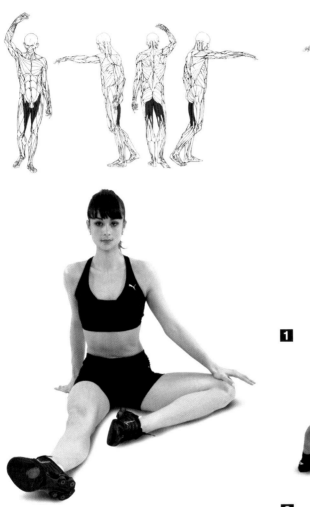

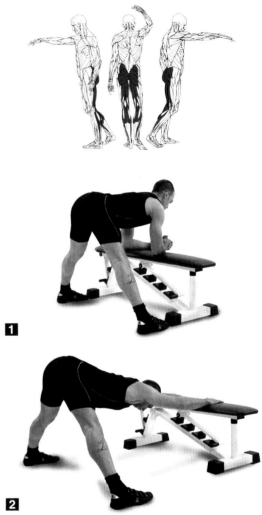

This exercise stretches the adductors in the bent leg as well as the hamstrings in the straight leg.

Sit in a tailor position with your back straight, your left leg bent, and your right leg straight out in front of you. Put your right hand on the floor behind you, keeping your arm straight. Put your left palm on your left knee and push gently to increase the stretch. Hold the stretch for 30 seconds while breathing slowly and regularly. Change sides and repeat the exercise.

This exercise stretches the adductors, buttocks, and hamstrings.

Stand by a bench with your legs as far apart as possible. Bend forward until your torso is horizontal. Put your forearms on the bench and clasp your hands. Hold the stretch for 30 seconds, breathing slowly and regularly throughout the exercise **1**. The wider apart you place your legs, the greater the stretch you will feel in the adductors. The more you lean forward, the greater the stretch you will feel in the hamstrings **2**.

SIDE LUNGE STRETCH
FOR ADDUCTORS AND HAMSTRINGS

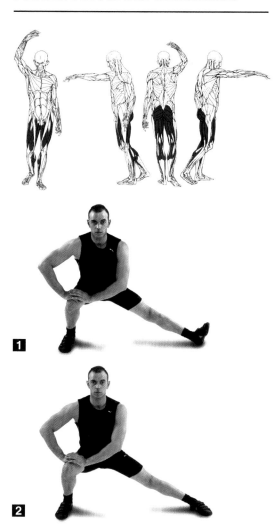

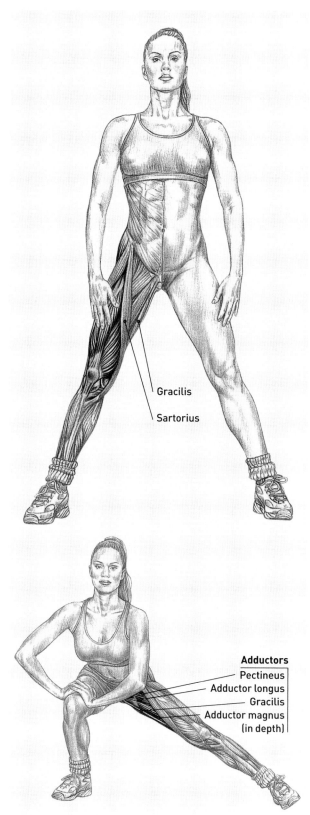

Gracilis

Sartorius

Adductors
Pectineus
Adductor longus
Gracilis
Adductor magnus
(in depth)

This exercise stretches the adductors, buttocks, and hamstrings.

From a standing position, do a lunge to the side. Clasp your hands and put them on the thigh of your bent leg just above the knee. If the tip of the foot on the straight leg is pointing up, this will stretch the adductors and hamstrings **1**. If the foot of the straight leg is on the floor, this will primarily stretch the adductors **2**. Hold your chosen position for 30 seconds while breathing slowly and regularly. Change sides and repeat the exercise.

STRETCHES FOR THE CALVES

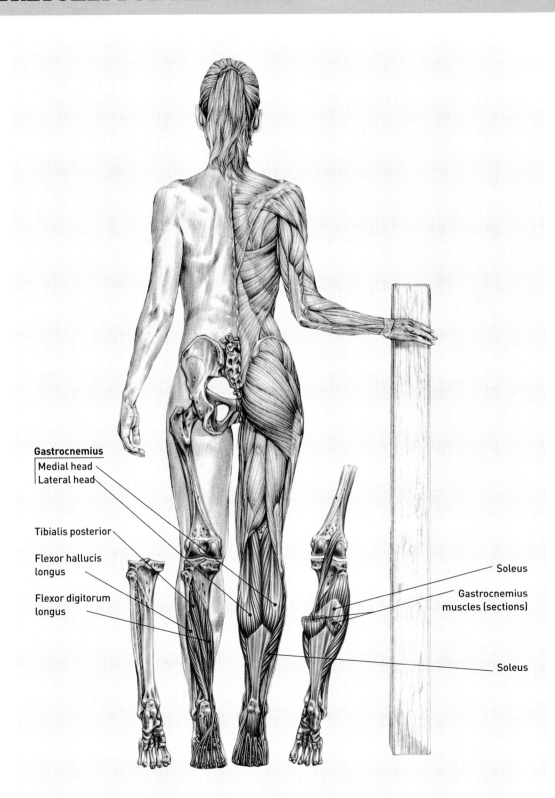

Gastrocnemius
Medial head
Lateral head

Tibialis posterior

Flexor hallucis longus

Flexor digitorum longus

Soleus

Gastrocnemius muscles (sections)

Soleus

Calf stretches have two purposes:

→ They keep the ankle flexible (over the years, this joint tends to become stiff).
→ They prevent twisted ankles, which can happen if you step awkwardly or if you run on uneven terrain.

Athletes, more than anyone else, should conscientiously stretch the calves to protect stride and to prevent injuries that so frequently happen to the ankles.

Note

Calf stretches can be done on a single leg or on both legs at the same time. The range of motion is much greater when you stretch a single leg, because you are always more flexible when stretching on only one side, and your body weight will force the stretch farther if it is pushing on only one leg rather than if it is distributed between both legs.

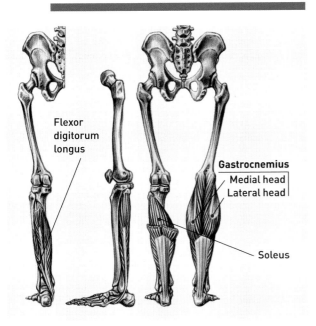

Flexor digitorum longus

Gastrocnemius
Medial head
Lateral head

Soleus

Always stretch your calves before any exercise!
To avoid twisting the ankle or damaging the Achilles tendon, you need to keep your feet very flexible. No matter what sport you play, your workouts should always begin with calf stretches. The calves are attached to the femurs. So to warm up the knee joint properly, stretch the calves before working the quadriceps or the hamstrings.

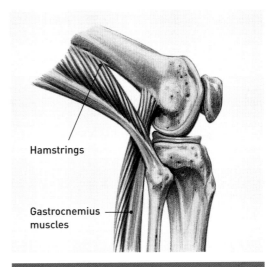

Hamstrings

Gastrocnemius muscles

Note

When you twist your ankle, you damage the ligaments that maintain the peroneus brevis and peroneus longus in their groove. Stretching and warming up these two muscles reduces the risk of injury.

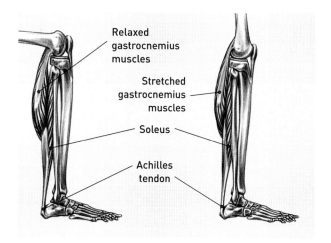

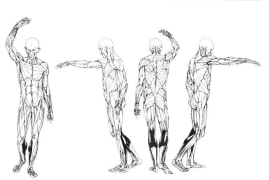

STRAIGHT-LEG CALF STRETCH

There are numerous ways to stretch your calves. When the leg is very straight, you are primarily stretching the gastrocnemius muscle. When the leg is bent, you are stretching the soleus. It is important to stretch the calves in a variety of ways (standing, in lunges, and by twisting) because each movement works on flexibility in a distinct part of the calf. These exercises are complementary.

Shoes or Bare Feet?

It is possible to be barefoot while stretching your calves. However, for the protection and comfort of the plantar aponeurosis, it is more sensible to wear athletic shoes, especially if you are an athlete. In fact, shoes allow your ankles to be in a normal position (as if on the floor). In addition, thanks to the comfort offered by shoes, you can go farther in a stretch so long as you are wearing flat shoes.

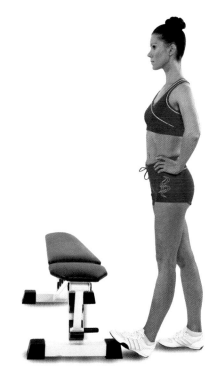

This exercise stretches the posterior calf muscle.

Stand with your torso straight and your hands on your waist. Contract your abdominal muscles and buttocks for better stability. Then put one leg forward and place the tip of the foot on a support a few inches high, but leave your heel on the floor. Hold this position for 30 seconds while breathing slowly and regularly. Change sides and repeat the exercise.

BENT-LEG CALF STRETCH

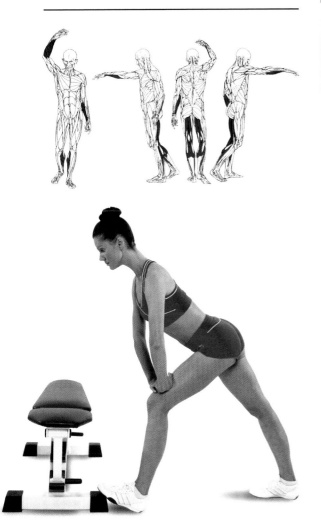

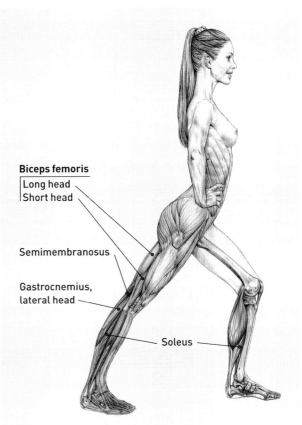

Biceps femoris
Long head
Short head

Semimembranosus

Gastrocnemius,
lateral head

Soleus

Stand with your hands on your waist and do a small lunge forward. Keep your torso very straight and your back leg straight behind you with the foot flat on the floor. Hold this position for 30 seconds while breathing slowly and regularly. Change sides and repeat the exercise.

This exercise stretches the calves and makes the thighs and hamstrings more flexible.
Stand and put one leg forward. Put the tip of the foot on a support a few inches high, but leave your heel on the floor. Bend your leg and lean your torso forward. Put both of your hands on your thigh, just above the knee. Keep the other leg straight behind you with the foot flat on the floor. Hold the stretch for 30 seconds while breathing slowly and regularly. Change sides and repeat the exercise.

CALF STRETCH IN A LUNGE

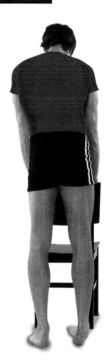

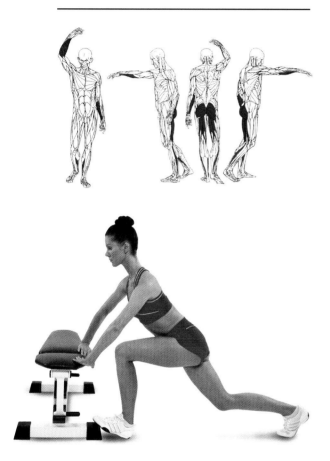

This exercise stretches the calves, thighs, buttocks, hamstrings, and hip flexors.
Do a forward lunge with a bench just in front of you. Put the tip of your forward foot on a support a few inches high, but keep your heel on the floor. Push both hands on the bench, and bend your back leg slightly while you raise the heel to increase the range of motion. Squeeze your abdominal muscles and your buttocks to keep your torso straight (be sure not to arch your back). Hold this position for 30 seconds while inhaling and exhaling slowly and regularly. Change sides and repeat the exercise.

Stand and support yourself with both hands on the back of a chair. Twist one foot to the side very slowly. Hold the stretch for about 15 seconds, then change feet. This version gives you greater control when stretching your ankles.

CALF AND ANKLE STRETCH

CONTROLLED VERSION

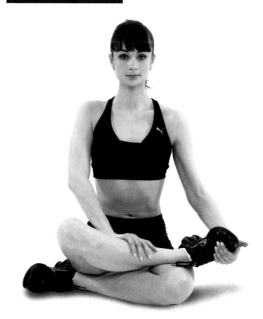

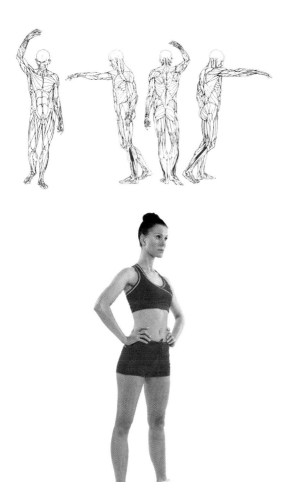

Sit on the floor with your torso straight, and put one bent leg on top of your other bent leg. Hold the top calf with one hand and grab the foot with the other hand. Gently pull upward to stretch the outside of the ankle. Hold the stretch for 30 seconds, then repeat the stretch on the other ankle. If you have stiff ankles, you can begin with this exercise. However, once your ankle is more flexible, this position will not generate enough natural tension to allow you to progress. At that point, you will need to move on to the previous exercise.

This exercise stretches the outside of the calves and ankles.
Stand and very slowly twist one of your feet to the side. Stabilize yourself with your other leg. Hold the stretch for 15 seconds, then change feet. We do not recommend, at least in the beginning, stretching both ankles at the same time. This will prevent any uncontrolled, and therefore excessive, stretching of the joint. This stretch is excellent for preventing sprained ankles.

STRETCHING PROGRAMS

STRETCHING PROGRAMS FOR BETTER MUSCLE TONE AND WELL-BEING

Here are three programs you can use to ease into stretching and become more familiar with the exercises.

BEGINNER PROGRAM

The beginner program should help make you more aware of your mobility. To rediscover your flexibility, do these exercises regularly.

To achieve the maximum benefit, you should

→ relax as much as you can,
→ be aware of your breathing,
→ be sure all of your muscles are getting enough oxygen,
→ let your muscle fibers relax gently, and
→ avoid jerky movements.

Note
Do all of the stretches described in each program in order with little rest time in between. This speed helps maintain your cardiovascular health while minimizing your total workout time. When you have done all the stretches in the program once, you will have completed a circuit. If necessary, repeat the circuit once or twice per session. We recommend that you do a circuit of these exercises twice weekly.

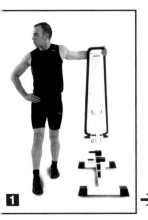

1

CHEST
p. 48
Time: 20 seconds per arm

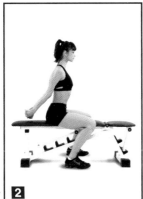

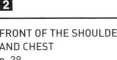

2

FRONT OF THE SHOULDER
AND CHEST
p. 39
Time: 30 seconds

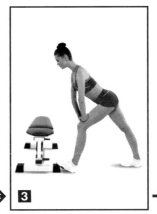

3

CALVES AND HAMSTRINGS
p. 123
Time: 20 seconds per leg

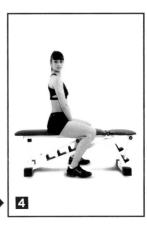

4

SIDE OF THE NECK
p. 32
Time: 30 seconds per side

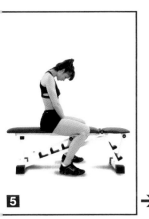

5

BACK OF THE NECK
p. 32
Time: 40 seconds

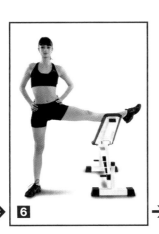

6

ADDUCTORS
AND HAMSTRINGS
p. 113
Time: 20 seconds per leg

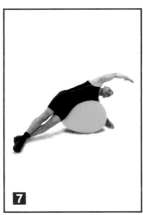

7

LATERAL FLEXORS
IN THE TORSO AND BACK
p. 61
Time: 20 seconds per side

INTERMEDIATE PROGRAM

Move on to this program once you feel well aware of your body's mobility, your breathing, and proper joint placement. In this program, hold the stretches longer to increase your range of motion. Inhale and exhale slowly and regularly throughout the stretches. We recommend that you do this program 2 or 3 times weekly and that you do 2 or 3 circuits per session.

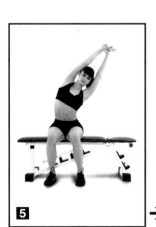

1

CALVES
p. 122
Time: 20 seconds per leg

→

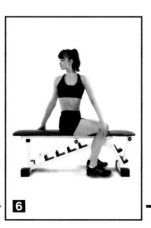

2

HAMSTRINGS, BUTTOCKS,
AND CALVES
p. 100
Time: 30 seconds per leg

→

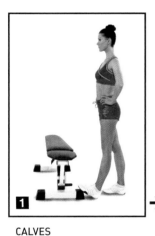

3

BUTTOCKS
AND HAMSTRINGS
p. 89
Time: 20 seconds per leg

→

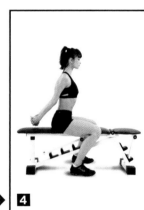

4

FRONT OF THE SHOULDER
AND CHEST
p. 39
Time: 30 seconds

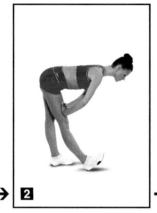

5

LATERAL FLEXORS
IN THE TORSO AND BACK
p. 60
Time: 20 seconds per side

→

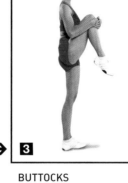

6

ROTATOR MUSCLES
IN THE TORSO
p. 64
Time: 30 seconds per side

→

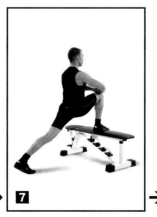

7

BUTTOCKS
AND HAMSTRINGS
p. 90
Time: 20 seconds per leg

→

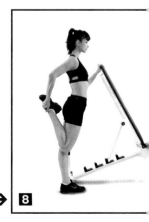

8

QUADRICEPS
p. 97
Time: 30 seconds per leg

ADVANCED PROGRAM

This program lets you master your body even more by working on placement details, especially in twisting and rotation. We recommend doing these exercises 3 or 4 times weekly and doing 3 to 5 circuits per session. If you are short on time, do half of the exercises in the morning and the other half in the evening.

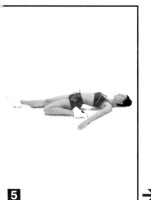 →

1

HIPS AND BUTTOCKS
p. 85
Time: 30 seconds per side

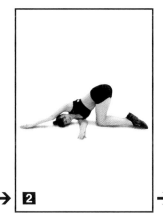 →

2

LATISSIMUS DORSI
AND ROTATOR MUSCLES
IN THE TORSO
p. 78
Time: 20 seconds per side

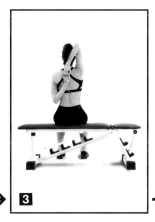 →

3

SHOULDER AND TRICEPS
p. 46
Time: 20 seconds per arm

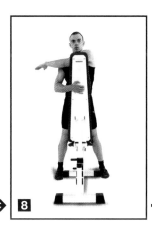 →

4

QUADRICEPS
p. 94
Time: 40 seconds

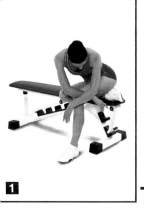 →

5

QUADRICEPS
p. 95
Time: 20 seconds per leg

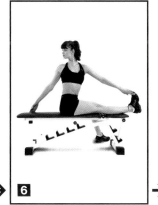 →

6

ROTATOR MUSCLES
IN THE TORSO
p. 66
Time: 30 seconds per side

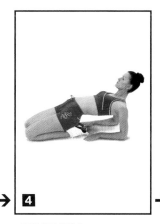 →

7

CHEST
p. 48
Time: 20 seconds per arm

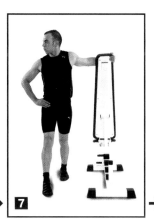 →

8

BACK OF THE SHOULDER
p. 45
Time: 45 seconds per arm

(continued)

Advanced Program *(continued)*

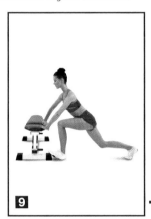

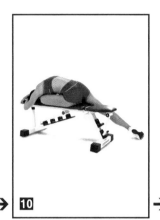

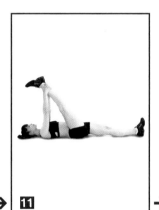

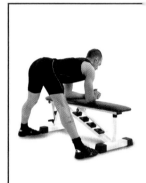

9

CALVES, HAMSTRINGS,
AND BUTTOCKS
p. 124
Time: **30 seconds per leg**

→

10

HIPS, BUTTOCKS,
AND BACK
p. 84
Time: **30 seconds per side**

→

11

HAMSTRINGS
AND PSOAS MUSCLES
p. 109
Time: **30 seconds per leg**

→

12

ADDUCTORS, BUTTOCKS,
AND HAMSTRINGS
p. 118
Time: **45 seconds**

STRETCHING PROGRAMS FOR ATHLETES

GUIDELINES FOR PROGRAMS

These programs are tailored to the specific needs of major sports. You must do these programs with gradually increasing intensity as you progress through your workout sessions. You should average about 2 sessions weekly. When you are satisfied that you have reached a certain level of flexibility, then 1 weekly session will be sufficient for maintaining that flexibility.

Do all of the stretches described in each program in order with little rest time in between. This speed helps maintain your cardiovascular health while minimizing your total workout time.

When you have done all the stretches in the program once, you will have completed a circuit. Repeat this circuit 2 or 3 times per session.

At first, you should hold each stretch for 15 to 45 seconds. Increase this time as you progress. Your objective is to reach 1 minute per exercise.

When you need to first stretch one side and then the other, begin on the right side during the first circuit. In the second circuit, start with the left side.

BASIC ATHLETIC PROGRAM

This basic program will quickly and easily increase flexibility in all of your joints. We recommend performing 3 to 5 circuits per session.

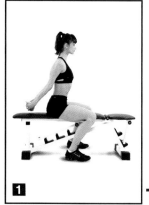

1

FRONT OF THE SHOULDER
AND CHEST
p. 39
Time: **40 seconds**

→

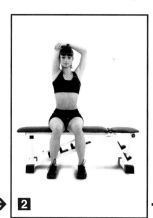

2

TRICEPS
p. 52
Time: **20 seconds per arm**

→

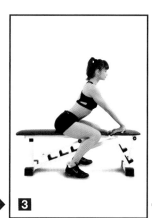

3

WRIST FLEXORS
p. 54
Time: **30 seconds**

→

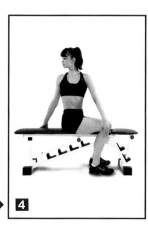

4

ROTATOR MUSCLES
IN THE TORSO
p. 64
Time: **30 seconds per side**

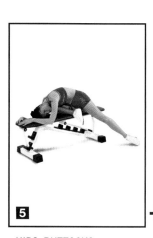

5

HIPS, BUTTOCKS,
AND BACK
p. 84
Time: **30 seconds per side**

→

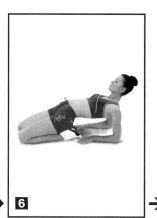

6

QUADRICEPS
p. 94
Time: **30 seconds**

→

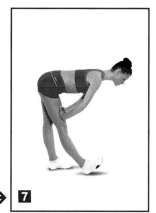

7

HAMSTRINGS, BUTTOCKS,
AND CALVES
p. 100
Time: **20 seconds per leg**

GOLF AND SPORTS INVOLVING TORSO ROTATION

The main objectives of this circuit are to increase the capacity to rotate the torso, protect the shoulders, and develop flexibility in the forearms. We recommend doing 4 to 6 circuits per session.

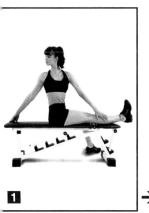

1

ROTATOR MUSCLES
IN THE TORSO
p. 65
Time: 30 seconds per side

→

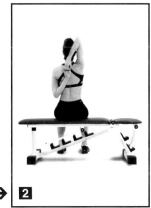

2

SHOULDER AND TRICEPS
p. 46
Time: 20 seconds per arm

→

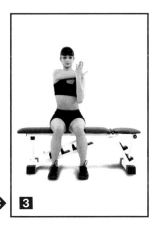

3

BACK OF THE SHOULDER,
TRAPEZIUS, AND
RHOMBOIDS
p. 43
Time: 20 seconds per arm

→

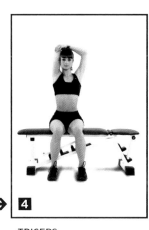

4

TRICEPS
p. 52
Time: 30 seconds per arm

→

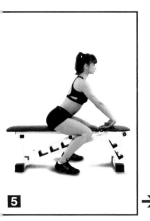

5

WRIST EXTENSORS
p. 56
Time: 30 seconds

→

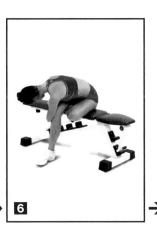

6

HIPS, BUTTOCKS,
AND BACK
p. 85
Time: 45 seconds per side

→

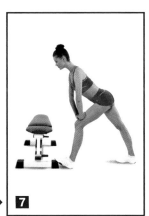

7

CALVES AND HAMSTRINGS
p. 123
Time: 30 seconds per leg

RUNNING SPORTS, SOCCER, AND SKATING

The primary objectives of this circuit are to prevent twisted ankles, develop flexibility in the hips, and increase the range of motion in all of the thigh muscles. We recommend doing 3 to 5 circuits per session.

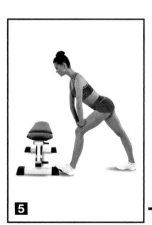

1

BUTTOCKS AND PSOAS
MUSCLES
p. 89
Time: **45 seconds per leg**

→

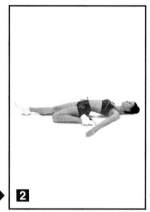

2

QUADRICEPS
p. 95
Time: **20 seconds per leg**

→

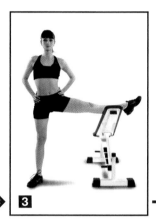

3

ADDUCTORS
AND HAMSTRINGS
p. 113
Time: **20 seconds per leg**

→

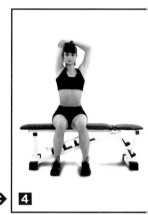

4

TRICEPS
p. 52
Time: **30 seconds per arm**

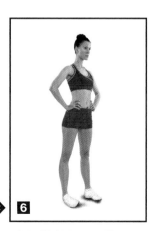

5

CALVES AND HAMSTRINGS
p. 123
Time: **20 seconds per leg**

→

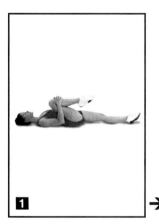

6

CALVES AND ANKLES
p. 125
Time: **45 seconds per leg**

SKIING

The primary objectives of this circuit are to increase the range of motion in all of the thigh muscles, prevent twisted ankles, and develop flexibility in the shoulders. We recommend doing 3 to 5 circuits per session.

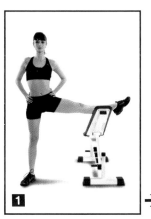

1

ADDUCTORS
AND HAMSTRINGS
p. 113
Time: **45 seconds per leg**

→

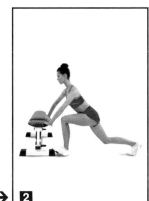

2

CALVES, HAMSTRINGS,
AND BUTTOCKS
p. 124
Time: **30 seconds per leg**

→

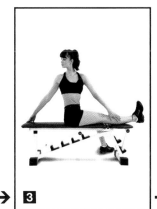

3

ROTATOR MUSCLES
IN THE TORSO
p. 65
Time: **45 seconds per side**

→

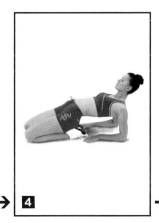

4

QUADRICEPS
p. 94
Time: **45 seconds per leg**

→

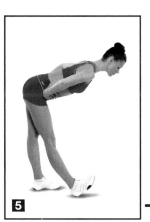

5

HAMSTRINGS, BUTTOCKS,
AND CALVES
p. 100
Time: **45 seconds per leg**

→

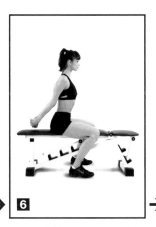

6

FRONT OF THE SHOULDER
AND CHEST
p. 39
Time: **45 seconds**

→

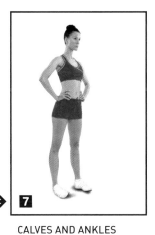

7

CALVES AND ANKLES
p. 125
Time: **45 seconds per leg**

COMBAT SPORTS

The primary objectives of this circuit are to increase mobility in the scapula, increase torso rotation, protect the neck, and increase range of motion in the lower body. We recommend doing 5 to 8 circuits per session.

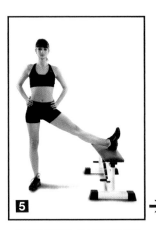

→

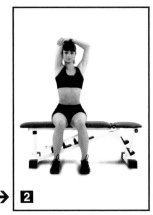

→

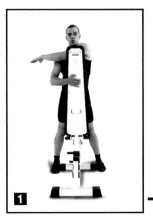

→

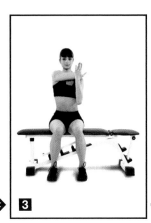

1 BACK OF THE SHOULDER
p. 45
Time: 45 seconds per arm

2 TRICEPS
p. 52
Time: 45 seconds per arm

3 BACK OF THE SHOULDER, TRAPEZIUS, AND RHOMBOIDS
p. 43
Time: 45 seconds per arm

4 ROTATOR MUSCLES IN THE TORSO
p. 66
Time: 45 seconds per side

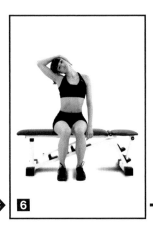

→

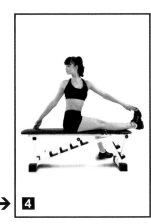

→

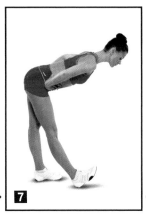

→

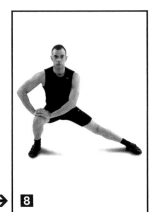

5 ADDUCTORS, HAMSTRINGS, AND CALVES
p. 112
Time: 45 seconds per leg

6 SIDE OF THE NECK
p. 30
Time: 45 seconds per side

7 HAMSTRINGS, BUTTOCKS, AND CALVES
p. 100
Time: 45 seconds per leg

8 ADDUCTORS, BUTTOCKS, AND HAMSTRINGS
p. 119
Time: 45 seconds per leg

CYCLING

The primary objectives of this circuit are to develop hip flexibility, increase the range of motion in the ankles, relax the shoulders, and stretch the back. We recommend doing 3 to 6 circuits per session.

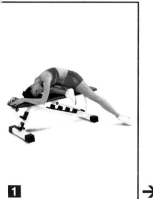

1

HIPS, BUTTOCKS,
AND BACK
p. 84
Time: 45 seconds per side

→

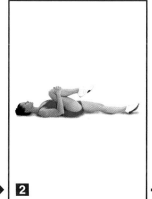

2

BUTTOCKS AND PSOAS
MUSCLES
p. 89
Time: 30 seconds per leg

→

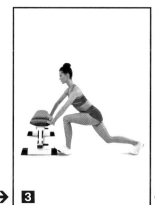

3

CALVES, HAMSTRINGS,
AND BUTTOCKS
p. 124
Time: 30 seconds per leg

→

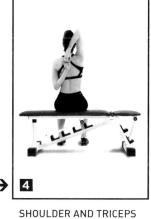

4

SHOULDER AND TRICEPS
p. 46
Time: 20 seconds per arm

→

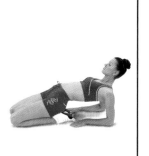

5

QUADRICEPS
p. 94
Time: 45 seconds

→

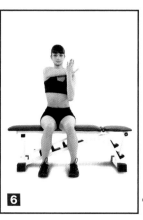

6

BACK OF THE SHOULDER,
TRAPEZIUS, AND
RHOMBOIDS
p. 43
Time: 20 seconds per arm

→

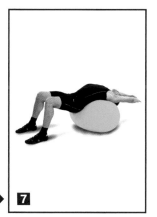

7

BACK AND ABDOMINAL
MUSCLES
p. 73
Time: 45 seconds

THROWING SPORTS
(SHOT PUT, BASKETBALL, AND HANDBALL)

The primary objectives of this circuit are to develop rotation in the torso, increase range of motion in the hip rotators, and protect the shoulders. We recommend doing 3 to 6 circuits per session.

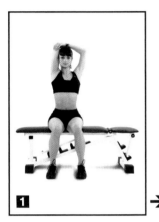 → 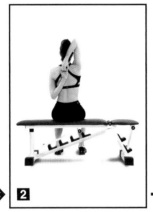 → 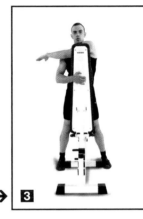 →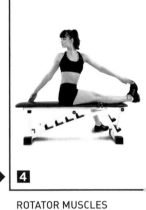

TRICEPS
p. 52
Time: 20 seconds per arm

SHOULDER AND TRICEPS
p. 46
Time: 15 seconds per arm

BACK OF THE SHOULDER
p. 45
Time: 20 seconds per arm

ROTATOR MUSCLES
IN THE TORSO
p. 66
Time: 45 seconds per side

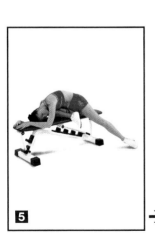 →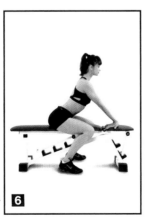

HIPS, BUTTOCKS,
AND BACK
p. 84
Time: 45 seconds per side

WRIST FLEXORS
p. 54
Time: 30 seconds

HORSEBACK RIDING

The primary objectives of this circuit are to develop flexibility in the hips, increase the range of motion in the adductors, decompress the spine, and relax the shoulders. We recommend doing 3 to 6 circuits per session.

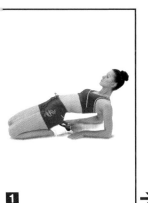

1

QUADRICEPS
p. 94
Time: 45 seconds

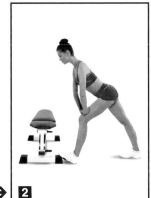

2

CALVES AND HAMSTRINGS
p. 123
Time: 30 seconds per leg

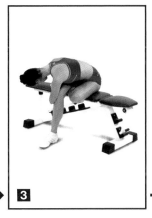

3

HIPS, BUTTOCKS,
AND BACK
p. 85
Time: 45 seconds per side

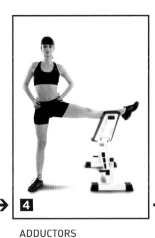

4

ADDUCTORS
AND HAMSTRINGS
p. 113
Time: 30 seconds per leg

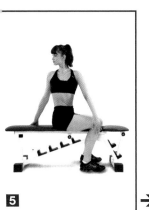

5

ROTATOR MUSCLES
IN THE TORSO
p. 64
Time: 45 seconds per side

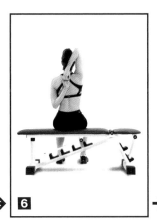

6

SHOULDER AND TRICEPS
p. 46
Time: 20 seconds per arm

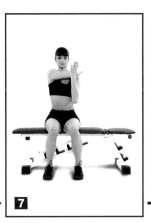

7

BACK OF THE SHOULDER,
TRAPEZIUS, AND
RHOMBOIDS
p. 43
Time: 20 seconds per arm

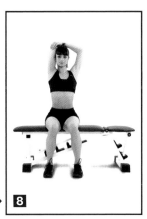

8

TRICEPS
p. 52
Time: 20 seconds per arm

SWIMMING

Champion swimmers have extraordinary flexibility, particularly in the shoulders, legs, and ankles as well as in the lumbar region. This is what you will achieve by using this program. We recommend doing 3 to 6 circuits per session.

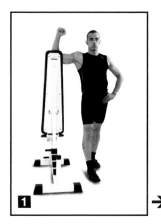

1

CHEST AND FRONT
OF SHOULDER
p. 47
Time: 30 seconds per side

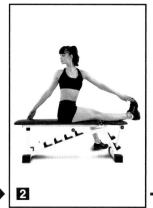

2

ROTATOR MUSCLES
IN THE TORSO
p. 66
Time: 45 seconds per side

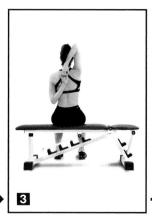

3

SHOULDER AND TRICEPS
p. 46
Time: 20 seconds per arm

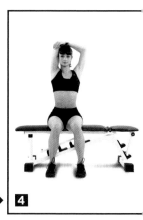

4

TRICEPS
p. 52
Time: 20 seconds per arm

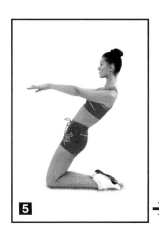

5

QUADRICEPS
p. 96
Time: 45 seconds

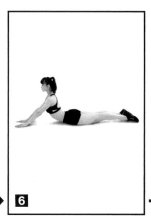

6

LUMBAR REGION AND
ABDOMINAL MUSCLES
p. 74
Time: 45 seconds

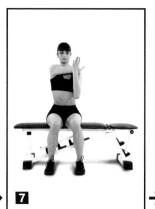

7

BACK OF THE SHOULDER,
TRAPEZIUS, AND
RHOMBOIDS
p. 43
Time: 20 seconds per arm

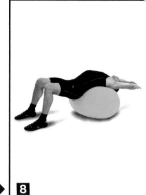

8

BACK AND ABDOMINAL
MUSCLES
p. 73
Time: 45 seconds

BODYBUILDING

More than any other activity, intense bodybuilding can reduce the range of motion in many joints. You can prevent this problem simply by following this stretching program regularly. Do this circuit at average intensity twice weekly at the end of your bodybuilding workout. In addition, stretch your spine by hanging from a fixed bar at the end of each workout. We recommend doing 2 to 4 circuits per session.

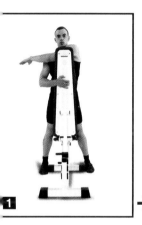 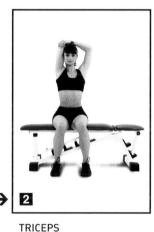 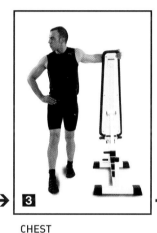 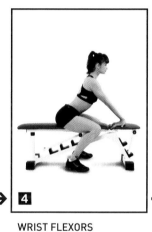

1
BACK OF THE SHOULDER
p. 45
Time: **20 seconds per arm**

2
TRICEPS
p. 52
Time: **20 seconds per arm**

3
CHEST
p. 48
Time: **30 seconds per arm**

4
WRIST FLEXORS
p. 54
Time: **30 seconds**

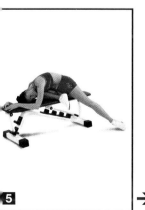 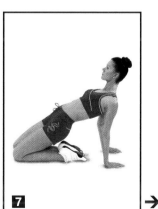 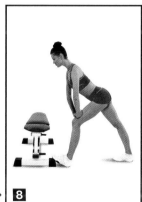 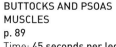

5
HIPS, BUTTOCKS,
AND BACK
p. 84
Time: **45 seconds per side**

6
BUTTOCKS AND PSOAS
MUSCLES
p. 89
Time: **45 seconds per leg**

7
QUADRICEPS
p. 94
Time: **45 seconds**

8
CALVES AND HAMSTRINGS
p. 123
Time: **30 seconds per leg**

Library of Congress Cataloging-in-Publication Data

Delavier, Frédéric.
 [Guide du stretching. English]
 Delavier's stretching anatomy / Frédéric Delavier, Jean-Pierre Clémenceau, Michael Gundill.
   p. cm.
 ISBN-13: 978-1-4504-1398-5 (soft cover)
 ISBN-10: 1-4504-1398-6 (soft cover)
 1. Stretching exercises. 2. Muscles--Anatomy. 3. Muscle strength. I. Clémenceau, Jean-Pierre. II. Gundill, Michael. III. Title. IV. Title
Stretching anatomy.
 RA781.63.D4513 2010
 613.7'1--dc22
                        2011009478

ISBN-10: 1-4504-1398-6 (print)
ISBN-13: 978-1-4504-1398-5 (print)

Copyright © 2010 by Éditions Vigot, 23 rue de l'École de Médecine, 75006 Paris, France

This publication is written and published to provide accurate and authoritative information relevant to the subject matter presented. It is published and sold with the understanding that the author and publisher are not engaged in rendering legal, medical, or other professional services by reason of their authorship or publication of this work. If medical or other expert assistance is required, the services of a competent professional person should be sought.

This book is a revised edition of *Guide du Stretching: Approche Anatomique Illustrée,* published in 2010 by Éditions Vigot.

Photography: © All rights reserved.
Illustrations: © All illustrations by Frédéric Delavier.
Graphics: Claire Guigal
Direction: Philippe Le Bihan
Publication: Chloé Chauveau
Photoengraving: Reproscan

Human Kinetics books are available at special discounts for bulk purchase. Special editions or book excerpts can also be created to specification. For details, contact the Special Sales Manager at Human Kinetics.

Printed in France - L58746A   10 9 8 7 6 5 4 3 2

Human Kinetics
Website: www.HumanKinetics.com

United States: Human Kinetics
P.O. Box 5076
Champaign, IL 61825-5076
800-747-4457
e-mail: humank@hkusa.com

Canada: Human Kinetics
475 Devonshire Road Unit 100
Windsor, ON N8Y 2L5
800-465-7301 (in Canada only)
e-mail: info@hkcanada.com

Europe: Human Kinetics
107 Bradford Road
Stanningley
Leeds LS28 6AT, United Kingdom
+44 (0) 113 255 5665
e-mail: hk@hkeurope.com

Australia: Human Kinetics
57A Price Avenue
Lower Mitcham, South Australia 5062
08 8372 0999
e-mail: info@hkaustralia.com

New Zealand: Human Kinetics
P.O. Box 80
Torrens Park, South Australia 5062
0800 222 062
e-mail: info@hknewzealand.com